FOR THE PUBLIC'S HEALTH
The Role of Measurement in Action and Accountability

D1409041

Committee on Public Health Strategies to Improve Health

Board on Population Health and Public Health Practice

INSTITUTE OF MEDICINE
OF THE NATIONAL ACADEMIES

THE NATIONAL ACADEMIES PRESS
Washington, D.C.
www.nap.edu

THE NATIONAL ACADEMIES PRESS   500 Fifth Street, N.W.   Washington, DC 20001

NOTICE: The project that is the subject of this report was approved by the Governing Board of the National Research Council, whose members are drawn from the councils of the National Academy of Sciences, the National Academy of Engineering, and the Institute of Medicine. The members of the committee responsible for the report were chosen for their special competences and with regard for appropriate balance.

This study was supported by Contract No. 65863 between the National Academy of Sciences and the Robert Wood Johnson Foundation. Any opinions, findings, conclusions, or recommendations expressed in this publication are those of the author(s) and do not necessarily reflect the view of the organizations or agencies that provided support for this project.

Library of Congress Cataloging-in-Publication Data

For the public's health : the role of measurement in action and accountability / Committee on Public Health Strategies to Improve Health, Board on Population Health and Public Health Practice, Institute of Medicine.
    p. ; cm.
Includes bibliographical references and index.
ISBN 978-0-309-16127-5 (hardcover : alk. paper) — ISBN 978-0-309-16128-2 (pdf : alk. paper) 1. Public health administration—United States. 2. Health status indicators—United States. I. Institute of Medicine (U.S.). Committee on Public Health Strategies to Improve Health.
    [DNLM: 1. Public Health Administration—standards—United States. 2. Health Status Indicators—United States. 3. Social Responsibility—United States. WA 540 AA1]
    RA445.F657 2011
    362.1—dc22
                            2011004593

Additional copies of this report are available from the National Academies Press, 500 Fifth Street, N.W., Lockbox 285, Washington, DC 20055; (800) 624-6242 or (202) 334-3313 (in the Washington metropolitan area); Internet, http://www.nap.edu.

For more information about the Institute of Medicine, visit the IOM home page at: www.iom.edu.

The serpent has been a symbol of long life, healing, and knowledge among almost all cultures and religions since the beginning of recorded history. The serpent adopted as a logotype by the Institute of Medicine is a relief carving from ancient Greece, now held by the Staatliche Museen in Berlin.

Suggested citation: IOM (Institute of Medicine). 2011. *For the Public's Health: The Role of Measurement in Action and Accountability.* Washington, DC: The National Academies Press.

"Knowing is not enough; we must apply.
Willing is not enough; we must do."
—Goethe

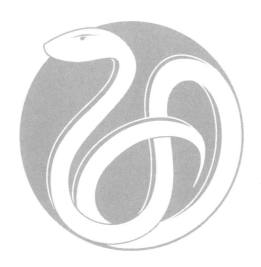

INSTITUTE OF MEDICINE
OF THE NATIONAL ACADEMIES

Advising the Nation. Improving Health.

THE NATIONAL ACADEMIES
Advisers to the Nation on Science, Engineering, and Medicine

The **National Academy of Sciences** is a private, nonprofit, self-perpetuating society of distinguished scholars engaged in scientific and engineering research, dedicated to the furtherance of science and technology and to their use for the general welfare. Upon the authority of the charter granted to it by the Congress in 1863, the Academy has a mandate that requires it to advise the federal government on scientific and technical matters. Dr. Ralph J. Cicerone is president of the National Academy of Sciences.

The **National Academy of Engineering** was established in 1964, under the charter of the National Academy of Sciences, as a parallel organization of outstanding engineers. It is autonomous in its administration and in the selection of its members, sharing with the National Academy of Sciences the responsibility for advising the federal government. The National Academy of Engineering also sponsors engineering programs aimed at meeting national needs, encourages education and research, and recognizes the superior achievements of engineers. Dr. Charles M. Vest is president of the National Academy of Engineering.

The **Institute of Medicine** was established in 1970 by the National Academy of Sciences to secure the services of eminent members of appropriate professions in the examination of policy matters pertaining to the health of the public. The Institute acts under the responsibility given to the National Academy of Sciences by its congressional charter to be an adviser to the federal government and, upon its own initiative, to identify issues of medical care, research, and education. Dr. Harvey V. Fineberg is president of the Institute of Medicine.

The **National Research Council** was organized by the National Academy of Sciences in 1916 to associate the broad community of science and technology with the Academy's purposes of furthering knowledge and advising the federal government. Functioning in accordance with general policies determined by the Academy, the Council has become the principal operating agency of both the National Academy of Sciences and the National Academy of Engineering in providing services to the government, the public, and the scientific and engineering communities. The Council is administered jointly by both Academies and the Institute of Medicine. Dr. Ralph J. Cicerone and Dr. Charles M. Vest are chair and vice chair, respectively, of the National Research Council.

www.national-academies.org

Reviewers

This report has been reviewed in draft form by individuals chosen for their diverse perspectives and technical expertise, in accordance with procedures approved by the National Research Council's Report Review Committee. The purpose of this independent review is to provide candid and critical comments that will assist the institution in making its published report as sound as possible and to ensure that the report meets institutional standards for objectivity, evidence, and responsiveness to the study charge. The review comments and draft manuscript remain confidential to protect the integrity of the deliberative process. We wish to thank the following individuals for their review of this report:

Edward Baker, University of North Carolina at Chapel Hill
Leah Devlin, University of North Carolina at Chapel Hill
Paul Erwin, University of Tennessee
Russ Glasgow, National Institutes of Health
Ron Z. Goetzel, Emory University
Anthony Iton, The California Endowment
Kenneth W. Kizer, Kizer & Associates, LLC
Paula M. Lantz, University of Michigan
Elizabeth A. McGlynn, The RAND Corporation
David Meltzer, University of Chicago
Margaret Potter, University of Pittsburgh
Mary Selecky, Washington State Department of Health
Burton H. Singer, University of Florida
Edward H. Wagner, Group Health Research Institute

Although the reviewers listed above have provided many constructive comments and suggestions, they were not asked to endorse the conclusions or recommendations nor did they see the final draft of the report before its release. The review of this report was overseen by **Lawrence D. Brown,** University of Pennsylvania, and **Jo Ivey Boufford,** New York University. Appointed by the National Research Council and the Institute of Medicine, they were responsible for making certain that an independent examination of this report was carried out in accordance with institutional procedures and that all review comments were carefully considered. Responsibility for the final content of this report rests entirely with the authoring committee and the institution.

Acknowledgments

The committee wishes to thank colleagues both outside and inside the National Academies who provided valuable information at various points in the study process. These include Connie Citro (National Research Council [NRC]), Gooloo Wunderlich (NRC), Michael Wolfson (University of Ottawa, formerly, Statistics Canada), and Jennifer Madans (National Center for Health Statistics, Centers for Disease Control and Prevention).

The committee learned a great deal about measurement of health from representatives of federal, state, and local public health agencies and from researchers and many types of practitioners who presented at the committee's information-gathering meetings pertaining to the present report. The meeting agendas provided in Appendix C include the names of all the speakers.

Additional support with one technical area of the report was provided by IBM Research Division colleagues of committee member Martín Sepúlveda. The committee thanks Peter Haas, Paul Maglio, and Pat Selinger for their assistance with report discussions about modeling.

Finally, the committee would also like to thank the Institute of Medicine staff members who contributed to the production of this report, including study staff Alina Baciu, Amy Geller, Alejandra Martín, Raina Sharma, Allison Berger, Rose Marie Martinez, and Hope Hare, as well as other staff on the Board on Population Health who provided occasional support. The project received valuable help from Norman Grossblatt (senior editor), Christine Stencel (Office of News and Public Information), Christie Bell and Amy Przybocki (Office of Financial Administration), and Greta Gorman and colleagues (IOM Office of Review and Communication).

Contents

Preface:
Introduction to the Series of Reports

In 2009, the Robert Wood Johnson Foundation asked the Institute of Medicine (IOM) to convene a committee to examine three topics in relation to public health: measurement, the law, and funding. The committee's complete three-part charge is provided in Box P-1. The IOM Committee on Public Health Strategies to Improve Health explored the topics in the context of contemporary opportunities and challenges and with the prospect of influencing the work of the health system (broadly defined as in the report summary) in the second decade of the 21st century and beyond. The committee was asked to prepare three reports—one on each topic—that contained actionable recommendations for public health agencies and other stakeholders that have roles in the health of the US population. This report is the first in the series.

The committee's three tasks and the series of reports prepared to respond to them are linked by the recognition that measurement, laws, and funding are three major drivers of change in the health system. Measurement (with the data that support it) helps specialists and the public to understand health status in different ways (for example, by determinant or underlying cause where national, local, and comparative evidence is available), to understand the performance of the various stakeholders in the system, and to understand the health-related results of investment. Measurement also helps communities to understand their current status, to determine whether they are making progress in improving health, and to set priorities for their next actions. Although the causal chains between actions of the health system and health outcomes are not always clearly elucidated, measurement is a fundamental requirement for the reasons listed above.

BOX P-1
Charge to the Committee

Task 1 (accomplished in this report)
The committee will review population health strategies, associated metrics, and interventions in the context of a reformed health care system. The committee will review the role of score cards and other measures or assessments in summarizing the impact of the public health system, and how these can be used by policy-makers and the community to hold both government and other stakeholders accountable and to inform advocacy for public health policies and practices.

Task 2 (to be addressed in a forthcoming report)
The committee will review how statutes and regulations prevent injury and disease, save lives, and optimize health outcomes. The committee will systematically discuss legal and regulatory authority; note past efforts to develop model public health legislation; and describe the implications of the changing social and policy context for public health laws and regulations.

Task 3 (to be addressed in a forthcoming report)
The committee will develop recommendations for funding state and local health systems that support the needs of the public after health care reform. Recommendations should be evidence based and implementable. In developing their recommendations the committee will:

- Review current funding structures for public health
- Assess opportunities for use of funds to improve health outcomes
- Review the impact of fluctuations in funding for public health
- Assess innovative policies and mechanisms for funding public health services and community-based interventions and suggest possible options for sustainable funding.

Laws transform the underpinnings of the health system and also act at various points in and on the complex environments that generate the conditions for health. Those environments include the widely varied policy context of multiple government agencies, such as education and transportation agencies, and many types of legal or legislative measure intended to reshape the factors that improve or impede health. The measures range from national tobacco policy to local smoking bans and from national agricultural subsidies and school nutrition standards to local school-board decisions about the types of foods and beverages to be sold in school vending machines.

Funding that supports the activities of public health agencies is provided primarily by federal, state, and local governments. However, government budgets must balance a variety of needs, programs, and policies, and the budgets draw on different sources (including different types of taxes and fees), depending on jurisdiction. Therefore, the funds allocated to public health depend heavily on how the executive and legislative branches set priorities. Other funding sources support public health activities in the community, including "conversion" foundations formed when nonprofit hospitals and health insurers became privatized (such as the California Wellness Foundation). Additionally, funds for population health and medical care activities may be provided by community-based organizations with substantial resources, not-for-profit clinical care providers, and stakeholders in other sectors.

The subjects addressed in the three reports are not independent of each other and often affect one another. For example, measurement of health outcomes and of progress in meeting objectives can provide evidence to guide the development and implementation of public health laws and the allocation of resources for public health activities. Laws and policies often require the collection of data and can circumscribe the uses to which the data are put (for example, prohibiting access to personally identifiable health information). Similarly, statutes can affect funding for public health through such mechanisms as program-specific taxes or fees. And laws shape the structure of public health agencies, grant them their authority, and influence policy.

In the three reports, the committee will make a case for increased accountability of all sectors that affect health—including the clinical care delivery system, the business sector, academe, nongovernment organizations, communities, and various government agencies—with coordination by the government public health infrastructure. The present report reflects the committee's thinking about how accountability would look at local, state, and national levels[1] and suggests measurement strategies that would heighten accountability and galvanize broader action by communities and other stakeholders. In later reports, the committee will review legal and regulatory strategies that heighten public and private responsibilities and, in the final report, will consider resource needs and approaches to addressing them in a sustainable manner to ensure a robust population health system.

---

[1] The committee's discussion about measurement framework for accountability may also apply to territorial and tribal government, although this is not explicitly stated.

Summary

For the Public's Health: The Role of Measurement in Action and Accountability, this first of three reports, builds on earlier Institute of Medicine (IOM) efforts to describe the activities and role of the public health system, which was defined in the 2003 report *The Future of the Public's Health in the 21st Century* (IOM, 2003) as the intersectoral system that comprises the government public health agencies and various partners, including communities, the health care delivery system, employers and business, the media, and academia. In the present report, the system has been redefined as simply "the health system." The modifiers *public* and *population* are poorly understood by most people other than public health professionals and may have made it easier to misinterpret or overlook the collective influence and responsibility that all sectors have for creating and sustaining the conditions necessary for health. In describing and using the term *the health system,* the committee seeks to reinstate the proper and evidence-based understanding of health as not merely the result of medical or clinical care but the result of the sum of what we do as a society to create the conditions in which people can be healthy (IOM, 1988).

The committee's charge in preparing this report was to "review population health strategies, associated metrics, and interventions in the context of a reformed health care system. The committee will review the role of score cards and other measures or assessments in summarizing the impact of the public health system, and how these can be used by policy-makers and the community to hold both government and other stakeholders accountable and to inform advocacy for public health policies and practices."[1] At the committee's first meeting, the sponsor clarified the intent of the reference to the "public health system" to mean the multisectoral system described in the 2003 IOM report rather than the government public health infrastructure alone (IOM, 2003).

This report is the committee's response to its first task and hence focuses on measurement and on the US health statistics and information system, which collects, analyzes, and reports population health data, clinical care data, and health-relevant information from other sectors. However, data and measures are not ends in themselves, but rather tools to inform the myriad activities (programs, policies, and processes) developed or undertaken by governmental public health agencies and their many partners, and the committee recognizes that its later reports on the law and funding will complete its examination of three of the key drivers of population health improvement.

The committee finds that the United States lacks a coherent template for population health information that could be used to understand the health status of Americans and to assess how well the nation's efforts and investments result in improved population health. The committee recommends changes in the processes, tools, and approaches used to gather information on health outcomes and to assess accountability. This report contains four chapters that offer seven recommendations relevant to public health agencies, other government agencies, decision-makers and policy-makers, the private sector, and the American public.

The national preoccupation with the cost of clinical care evident in the lead-up to the passage of the Affordable Care Act of 2010 is well founded, and changes in the system's pricing, labor, processes, and technology are essential and urgent (see Chapter 1). However, improving the clinical care delivery system's efficiency and effectiveness will probably have only modest effects on the health of the population overall in the absence of an ecologic, population-based approach to health improvement. Unhealthy communities and unfavorable socioeconomic environments will continue to facilitate unhealthy choices and unhealthy environments.

The expected reform of the clinical care delivery system and the committee's understanding of the centrality of socioenvironmental determinants of health led it to view measures of health outcomes (often presented as indicators for public or policy-maker consumption and conveying statistical data directly or in a composite form) as serving three primary functions:

---

[1] Although the committee uses *clinical care system* in the report to refer to the health care or medical care delivery system, the language in this quotation comes directly from the sponsor's charge to the committee, so it was not changed.

- To provide transparent and easily understood information to members of communities and the public and private entities that serve them about health and the stakeholders that influence it locally and nationally.
- To galvanize and promote participation and responsibility on the part of the public and institutional stakeholders (businesses, employers, community members, and others) that have roles to play in improving population health.
- To foster greater accountability for performance in health improvement on the part of government health agencies, other government entities whose portfolios have direct bearing on the health of Americans, and private-sector and nonprofit-sector contributors to the health system.

The committee believes that analysis and use of health and relevant nonhealth data and measures are a necessary complement to and facilitator of other efforts in the transformation to healthier people, healthier community environments, and a strong, competitive national economy. Achieving those outcomes relies on an integration and building of synergy between the best evidence-based interventions at the population level and in the clinical setting. Measurement of health outcomes and performance can spur change—as demonstrated by communities that have been able to "move the needle" in their own local efforts to improve the conditions for health and in the clinical care system's efforts to improve quality.

More complete, useful, timely, and geographically pertinent information is a necessary but not sufficient ingredient to facilitate heightened community engagement and improved performance by various stakeholders in the health system, defined as encompassing the "activities undertaken within the formal structure of government and the associated efforts of private and voluntary organizations and individuals" (IOM, 1988, 2003).

In Chapter 1, the committee constructs its case for change that will lead to a transformed health statistics and information system and to a more concrete framework for placing measurement in the service of accountability. The committee's case includes an overview of the literature on the determinants of health and implications for the issues discussed in the remainder of the report.

In Chapter 2, the committee discusses the national health statistics and information enterprise. That enterprise is large and productive, but it lacks optimal coordination, it has gaps that impede its contributions to understanding of and improvement in population health outcomes, it does not shed sufficient light on the relevance of the determinants of health nationally or in communities, and it does not sufficiently inform about how the nation or communities can achieve improvements in health apart from those provided by traditional public health programs and by clinical care. For example, such health outcomes as infant mortality and cardiovascular disease expose the limits of a national health strategy that directs the vast majority of its resources toward change in the clinical care delivery system without equally aggressive attacks on the loci of conditions that lead to the adoption of unhealthy behaviors and creation of unhealthy environments. Without understanding and acting on those important conditions that can improve people's ability to live healthy lives, the United States will continue to incur needless clinical care costs, and the health of the population will fall further behind that of other nations.

In Chapter 3, the committee offers a series of recommendations to address the challenges described in Chapter 2, beginning with a transformation of the nation's primary health statistics agency. The transformation, the committee believes, has the potential to improve system-wide coordination and capacity to ensure that needed data are available to health-system partners. That is, to ensure that the best evidence is built through research and modeling to facilitate effective, efficient, and equitable actions to improve population health. The chapter's other recommendations are for the development and adoption of three types of measures that could better inform the public, decision-makers, public health practitioners, and their many partners about health outcomes and their determinants; an annual report on the socioeconomic determinants of health; modeling for predictive and systems use; data-sharing between public health agencies and medical care organizations; and public health agency reporting on clinical care performance pertinent to population health.

In Chapter 4, the committee uses the lens of measurement to examine and discuss system performance. It reviews the responsibilities of all stakeholders in the health system and outlines a framework for defining accountability and holding stakeholders accountable for the contributions they can make to population health. At the end of the chapter, the committee envisions what could happen in a transformed, high-performance health system in which the capacities of local laws, workplace policies, business decisions, clinical encounters, and public participation are harnessed to achieve marked gains in two exemplar health outcomes in individuals and communities: infant mortality and cardiovascular disease.

RECOMMENDATIONS

The committee finds that at all levels of American life—including local, state, and national—decision-makers lack sufficient information to make important choices about the health of their communities. That is due in part to the lack of sufficient coordination, integration, coherence, and capacity of the complex, multisectoral health statistics and information enterprise that generates, analyzes, and translates pertinent information for decision-makers and the public. The report's first recommendation proposes a solution.

Recommendation 1
The committee recommends that:
1. **The Secretary of Health and Human Services transform the mission of the National Center for Health Statistics to provide leadership to a renewed population health information system through enhanced coordination, new capacities, and better integration of the determinants of health.**
2. **The National Prevention, Health Promotion, and Public Health Council include in its annual report to Congress on its national prevention and health-promotion strategy an update on the progress of the National Center for Health Statistics transformation.**

The committee finds that the nation's population health statistics and information enterprise lacks three types of measures that could support the information needs of policy-makers, public health officials, health system partners, and communities. These are: a standardized set of measures that can be used to assess the intrinsic health of communities in and of themselves; a standardized set of health outcome indicators for national, state, and local use; and a summary measure of population health that can be used to estimate and track health-adjusted life expectancy (HALE)[2] for the United States. To elaborate on each of the measures, despite a long history of efforts to develop and implement the summary measure of population health in national data sets, such as National Center for Health Statistics (NCHS) surveys and the Healthy People objectives, no summary measure appropriate for calculating HALE has been adopted for routine use by federal agencies. Also, there currently is no coordinated, standard set of true measures of a community's health—not aggregated information about the health of individuals residing in a community, but rather measures of green space, availability of healthy foods, land use and zoning practices that are supportive of health, safety, social capital, and social cohesion, among many other determinants of health. Finally, the committee notes a proliferation of health outcome indicator sets (measures of distal health

---

[2] A definition of health-adjusted life expectancy (HALE): "Year-equivalents of full health that an individual can expect to live if exposed at each age to current mortality and morbidity patterns. Years of less than full health are weighted according to severity of health conditions. The HALE calculation modifies a standard life expectancy calculation by weighting the number of life years lived by each age group using the mean health state score for that age group" (Statistics Canada, 2006). Additional discussion of HALE and of summary measures of population health is provided in Chapter 3.

outcomes such as disease rates and disease-specific death rates), some of high quality, and all designed for different purposes but with a degree of overlap and the potential to cause confusion among decision-makers. The committee was not constituted to and did not endeavor to develop lists of proposed indicators. The process of developing and reaching evidence-based consensus on standardized indicator sets will require considerable research, broad-based discussion (involving all relevant parties), and priority-setting to come up with parsimonious sets. Research would include modeling and other efforts to elucidate the linked nature of many determinants of health and intermediate indicators of health. Clarifying those relationships can lead to development of useful measures at all geographic levels. A national effort toward such elucidation may initially require defining a modest core set that all localities would be encouraged to use (for example, to support comparisons and allow "rolling up" from the local to the state and even national levels); additional optimal indicators could be identified for other outcomes or community characteristics of interest to particular localities.

Recommendation 2
The committee recommends that the Department of Health and Human Services support and implement the following to integrate, align, and standardize health data and health-outcome measurement at all geographic levels:
a. **A core, standardized set of indicators that can be used to assess the health of communities.**
b. **A core, standardized set of health-outcome indicators for national, state, and local use.[3]**
c. **A summary measure of population health that can be used to estimate and track health-adjusted life expectancy for the United States.**

Ideally, the development of the indicators described above will be conducted with advice from a fully resourced and strengthened NCHS (see Recommendation 1) and input from other relevant stakeholders, including other agencies and organizations that collect, analyze, and report data; community-level public health practitioners; and the public health research community.

Because the summary measure of population health in part (c) would serve as a marker of the progress of the nation and its communities in improving health, it should be implemented in data-collection and public-communication efforts at the federal level (such as the periodic Healthy

---

[3] The conception of a community may differ from one context to another, and it could range from a neighborhood to a county. Local decision-makers may include mayors, boards of supervisors, and public health officials. The notion of local may also vary (from census tract or ZIP code to city or county) depending on planning or research objectives and many other factors.

People effort, which as discussed in Chapter 3 has attempted to include such a summary measure in the past) and at state and local levels. The committee believes that public officials need to take steps to educate Americans with respect to the meaning of summary measures of population health and their linkage to determinants that are amenable to action at individual and societal levels. Promotion of and education on the summary measure of population health will be needed if it is to can gain traction as a key marker of the progress of the nation and its communities in improving health.

Many commentators in the field have expressed great expectations about the potential of health-information technology, such as electronic health records, to inform population health activities and public health practice, and the Affordable Care Act calls for investment to inform public health and population health data-gathering. However, great care is needed to ensure that new investment meets all the stated goals, is not used largely to maximize the use and usefulness of clinical care data in the care delivery system in isolation from population health stakeholders, and gives high priority to accuracy and safeguarding of confidentiality and privacy.

Despite broad recognition in health circles of the vital importance of nonclinical determinants of health in shaping population health, the committee has found that the United States does not have a centralized federal comprehensive annual report that highlights and tracks progress on the root causes of poor health at the population level. A newly strengthened and adequately resourced NCHS may be well suited to assume that responsibility.

Recommendation 3
The committee recommends that the Department of Health and Human Services produce an annual report to inform policy-makers, all health-system sectors, and the public about important trends and disparities in social and environmental determinants that affect health.

The committee was asked to consider the implications of health care reform for population health and for the public health infrastructure in the context of measurement. It is unclear what effects the Affordable Care Act will have on public health agencies' role in the delivery of clinical services. However, the committee found that the Affordable Care Act's emphasis on prevention and its other population health–oriented provisions offer an opportunity to consider ways to integrate clinical care and public health efforts to contribute to improving population health.

Both clinical care and public health stakeholders need to benefit from the data-sharing relationship. For example, clinicians need easier access to the data that they submit to government entities, access to analyses to help them to improve the appropriateness of the care they deliver, and access to other population health data (such as disparities and determinants) pertinent to the health status of the communities they serve and how they compare with the larger population so that they can tailor clinical care, outreach, and community services to meet needs better and improve outcomes. Similarly, clinical care system data have been shown to be an important source of syndromic surveillance information for infectious diseases, small-area health data, and service use patterns to inform population health efforts, including filling gaps in data available from other sources (NCVHS, 2010).

Recommendation 4
The committee recommends that governmental public health agencies partner with medical care organizations and providers in their jurisdictions to share information[4] derived from clinical-data sources, when appropriate, to inform relevant population health priorities. Such information will support core health indicators that are otherwise unavailable at some or all geographic levels.

The committee also believes that public health agencies can play an important role in reporting to the public on clinical care system performance. They already do to some extent in various states and jurisdictions with regard to specific services and care settings. There are important concerns about confidentiality and privacy that must be weighed along with the value of open disclosure and analysis. However, much more could be communicated to the public in an easy-to-understand format and in the context of a broader effort to inform and educate the public about effectiveness and efficiency in clinical care and to improve patients' decision-making.

Recommendation 5
The committee recommends that state and local public health agencies in each state collaborate with clinical care delivery systems to assure that the public has greater awareness of the appropriateness, quality, safety, and efficiency of clinical care services delivered in their state and community. Local performance reports about overuse, underuse, and misuse should be made available for selected interventions (including preventive and diagnostic tests, procedures, and treatment).

Chapter 2 highlights both the extraordinary capabilities of the population health statistics and information available to support population health

---

[4] Information shared will generally be deidentified and aggregated. In some circumstances, however, the data are and must be tracked individually (for example, for infectious-disease reporting and immunization-registry purposes). Variations in local needs and public health authority may lead to other types of data-use agreements.

improvement activities and the substantial gaps that remain. Gaps include an understanding of some of the more recently conceptualized and studied complex causal and interrelated pathways to health outcomes, such as the contributions of social cohesion. The gaps make the work of decision-makers and communities more difficult because they lack information needed to support policy-making, health-needs priority-setting, resource allocation, and other aspects of planning. The committee believes that an array of modeling techniques can help to fill knowledge gaps, advance the state of the science, and provide better and more timely information to decision-makers and stakeholders.

Recommendation 6
The committee recommends that the Department of Health and Human Services (HHS) coordinate the development and evaluation and advance the use of predictive and system-based simulation models to understand the health consequences of underlying determinants of health. HHS should also use modeling to assess intended and unintended outcomes associated with policy, funding, investment, and resource options.

The committee concludes that an accountability framework is needed that includes (1) reaching agreement among health-system stakeholders and those holding them accountable on specific plans of action for targeting health priorities; (2) holding implementing agencies or stakeholders accountable for execution of the agreed-on plans; and (3) measuring execution and outcomes and agreeing on a revised plan of action (an iterative loop). Chapter 4 highlights two types of accountability: contract accountability, referring to the financial and statutory relationships between government public health agencies (and to a smaller extent nonprofit public health organizations) and their funders; and compact accountability (or mutual accountability), referring to the agreement-based relationships among other stakeholders and with the community.

Recommendation 7
The committee recommends that the Department of Health and Human Services work with relevant federal, state, and local public-sector and private-sector partners and stakeholders to
1. Facilitate the development of a performance-measurement system that promotes accountability among governmental and private-sector organizations that have responsibilities for protecting and improving population health at local, state, and national levels. The system should include measures of the inputs contributed by those organizations (e.g., capabilities, resources, activities, and

programs) and should allow tracking of impact on intermediate and population health outcomes.

2. Support the implementation of the performance measurement system by
   a. Educating and securing the acceptance of the system by policy-makers and partners.
   b. Establishing data-collection mechanisms needed to construct accountability measures at appropriate intervals at local, state, and national levels.
   c. Encouraging early adoption of the system by key government and nongovernmental public health organizations and use of the system for performance reporting, quality improvement, planning, and policy development.
   d. Assessing and developing the necessary health-system capacity (e.g., personnel, training, technical resources, and organizational structures) for broader adoption of the framework, including specific strategies for steps to address nonperformance by accountable agencies and organizations.

Strategies to address nonperformance could (depending on the stakeholder) range from technical assistance, training, and mentorship to direct oversight and assumption of responsibilities and from consolidation with other jurisdictions (or regionalization) to pooling of resources or sharing of specific resources and expertise to increase agency capacity and meet performance standards to ensure that every person in every jurisdiction has access to a full set of public health services. Such strategies would be applied in a stepwise fashion that builds capacity locally and improves the health of the community.

CONCLUSION

The first decade of the 21st century has been an extremely active and productive time for health-outcome and other types of indicators. Multiple organizations have drawn on federal and other government data to derive or develop myriad indicators of the various dimensions of population health—from distal outcomes to underlying and intermediate causal factors. However, the proliferation of indicator sets (varied in quality and purpose) has the potential to create confusion and further fragmentation in a field that is already splintered among numerous public, private, and nonprofit producers, translators, conveyors, and users of data.

The committee has examined the role of data and indicators in informing action and creating accountability and has offered recommendations that if implemented can lead to a more coherent, efficient, and useful health information system. The changes and challenges of the future, ranging from an aging population to economic hardship, require a system that fully integrates the determinants of health perspective into its instruments and methods, that uses the benefits of new technologies to their fullest advantage to increase efficiency and maximize resources, and that builds information bridges among sectors. Finally, the health information system must be intensely focused on the needs of end users (communities and decision-makers at all geographic levels), engaging them in the evolution of efforts toward coherence, standardization, and rationalization of a measurement capacity that advances the health of the public.

REFERENCES

IOM (Institute of Medicine). 1988. *The Future of Public Health*. Washington, DC: National Academy Press.
IOM. 2003. *The Future of the Public's Health in the 21st Century*. Washington, DC: The National Academies Press.
NCVHS (National Committee on Vital and Health Statistics). 2010. *Toward Enhanced Information Capacities for Health: An NCVHS Concept Paper*. Washington, DC: HHS.
Statistics Canada. 2006. *Population Health Impact of Disease in Canada (PHI): Glossary*. http://www.phac-aspc.gc.ca/phi-isp/glossary-eng.php (November 2, 2010).

1

Introduction

The national dialogue leading to the passage of the Affordable Care Act of 2010 (ACA)[1] vetted the failure of world-class clinical care to deliver world-class population health outcomes and health equity. The opportunities for change facilitated by the new law can come to fruition only if accompanied by a strong and comprehensive national effort to implement a population-level approach to health across the spectrum of medical, social, and environmental determinants of health.

The United States spent 17.3 percent ($2.5 trillion) of its gross domestic product (GDP) on clinical care in 2009, a proportion exceeding that of any other industrialized nation (Truffer et al., 2010). Organisation for Economic Co-operation and Development (OECD) comparisons show a persisting US per capita cost for clinical care more than twice that of the next-highest-spending country in the world (OECD, 2009). For the most recent year reported, 2008, the United States spent $7,290 per capita (16 percent of GDP) on clinical care compared with an average of $2,934 (9 percent of GDP) in OECD countries (OECD, 2009). More detailed information about clinical care costs to employers and workers for those who receive medical insurance through their employer is provided in Box 1-1.

The outlook for American spending on clinical care in the next decade is sobering. Expenditures are projected to rise sharply to 19.3 percent ($4.5 trillion) of GDP by 2019 (Truffer et al., 2010) and to 34 percent of GDP

---

[1] "The comprehensive health care reform law was enacted in two parts: The Patient Protection and Affordable Care Act was signed into law in March 23, 2010[,] and was amended by the Healthcare and Education Reconciliation Act on March 30, 2010. The name 'Affordable Care Act' is used to refer to the final amended version of the law" (HealthCare.gov, 2010).

BOX 1-1
Clinical Care Costs for Employers and Workers

At the employee and employer levels, US clinical care system costs are exceedingly high and increasing at unsustainable rates relative to wages. In the 9-year period 1999–2007, average annual percentage increases in private health expenditures exceeded average annual percentage increases in wages by nearly a factor of 3 (Kaiser Family Foundation and Health Research and Educational Trust, 2007). From 1999 to 2009, the average premium for family health insurance and worker contributions rose by 131%, from $5,790 to $13,375 (Kaiser Family Foundation and Health Research and Eductional Trust, 2009). The individual portion of the premium rose from $1,543 to $3,515, and the employer portion rose from $4,247 to $9,860. In addition, workers saw a 47% cumulative increase in their out-of-pocket expenses for covered services during almost the same period, 2000–2008 (Commonwealth Fund, 2009).

Employers, like workers, are staggering under the weight of health care costs. Coupled with projected spending increases in excess of 6% over the succeeding decade (Truffer et al., 2010), US corporations face enormous global competitive pressures in labor cost, particularly from lower-wage rapid-growth countries. In 2009, the Business Roundtable, an organization composed of the chief executive officers of leading US corporations, projected a 166% increase on a per-employee basis over the next decade if existing annual rates of increases in health care costs persist during this period (Hewitt Associates, 2009).

by 2040 (Executive Office of the President, Council of Economic Advisers, 2009). From 2009 to 2019, individual costs for health-insurance coverage are projected to rise an average of 5.1 percent per year and out-of-pocket expenses 4.8 percent per year (Truffer et al., 2010).

The individual and population health return on those substantial clinical care expenditures is inadequate. In its 2008 *National Scorecard on U.S. Health System Performance*, the Commonwealth Fund reported on 37 indicators of performance spanning access, quality, efficiency, equity, and healthy lives (Davis et al., 2008). The report uses benchmarks from top-performing countries, U.S. states, regions, and health plans. In 2008, the US health system achieved an overall score of 65 compared with a possible 100. It ranked unfavorably on numerous indicators, including measures of mortality (such as infant mortality), effective and coordinated care (such as screening rates and hospital readmissions), patient-centered and timely care, access problems due to cost, and efficiency (for example, Medicare costs for chronic disease and emergency-room use for nonurgent conditions). US clinical care system performance on equity demonstrated numerous outcome disparities in risk ratios for selected measures, comparing those with high and low incomes, comparing whites with Hispanics or blacks, and comparing insured with uninsured persons (Doty and Holmgren, 2006; Schoen et al., 2008). In a 2010 update of the scorecard, US clinical care system performance was compared with that of Australia, Canada, Germany, the Netherlands, New Zealand, and the United Kingdom. The US clinical care system ranked last or next-to-last in all five dimensions of high-performance examined (access, quality, cost, equity, and healthy lives) (Davis et al., 2010).

The national preoccupation with the cost of clinical care is well founded, and the need for change is urgent. However, improving the clinical care delivery system's efficiency and effectiveness will probably have only a modest effect on the overall health of the population (see McGinnis and Foege, 1993; Woolf et al., 2010). Some effort has been made to estimate the preventable mortality (the rate of death due to all preventable causes, such as behaviors and environmental exposures, excluding largely unavoidable factors, such as genetics) that could be attributed to "shortfalls in medical care" (McGinnis et al., 2002). Although more work is needed to estimate the contributions of this and the other determinants of health, clinical care appears to explain only a portion of preventable mortality (see, for example, Nolte and McKee, 2008; Woolf et al., 2007).[2] For example, McGinnis and colleagues (2002) estimated that 10–15 percent of preventable mortality could be reduced by improvements in the availability or quality of clinical care. A complementary way to measure the effect of various factors on population outcomes is to consider changes in life expectancy (for example, departures from the baseline provided by annual US statistics on life expectancy at birth). A Department of Health and Human Services report found that about 5 of the 30 years of increased life expectancy realized by Americans in the 20th century could be attributable to better clinical care (HHS et al., 1994). Cutler and colleagues (2006) estimated that as much as 50 percent of life-expectancy gains could be ascribed to advances in clinical care. Even if the 50 percent gains were validated, substantial gains are to be found outside the clinical care system.[3]

The ACA put into motion processes for comprehensive reform of the clinical care system in the United States (HHS, 2010a). Major reform objectives in the act dealt with broadening clinical-insurance coverage, reforming insurance practices, and improving aspects of the delivery of clinical care. The act also offers an opportunity to integrate parts of clinical care and public health efforts better to improve population health in

---

[2] Woolf and colleagues (2007) conducted an analysis and examined the literature on the contribution of education to preventing death and found that improvements in educational status could have dramatic effects on health outcomes.

[3] See Booske and colleagues (2009) for a brief discussion of some of the literature and how it has been used to assign weights to determinants of health.

BOX 1-2
Provisions of the Patient Protection and Affordable Care Act and the Health Care and Education Affordability Reconciliation Act (Jointly, the Affordable Care Act [ACA])

Several ACA provisions are focused on prevention and wellness, including

(1) Establishment of a National Prevention, Health Promotion and Public Health Council to bring together many of the executive branch cabinet secretaries to strategize about the potential health impact of policies and programs in areas of government not explicitly concerned with health or charged with assuring population health,[a] and development of a National Prevention and Health Promotion Strategy (National Prevention Health Promotion and Public Health Council, 2010).

(2) Key National Indicators Initiative and Council to
   1. conduct comprehensive oversight of the newly established key national indicator system;
   2. make recommendations on how to improve the key national indicator system;
   3. coordinate with federal government users and information providers to assure access to relevant and quality data; and
   4. enter into contracts with the National Academy of Sciences (to help establish a key national indicator system, by either creating its own institutional capability, or partnering with an independent, private, non-profit organization; identify and select all criterion and methodologies to establish and operate the key national indicator system; design, publish, and maintain a public website for

the United States—actions ranging from improved delivery of effective clinical preventive services to population-based interventions that include broad changes in the many dimensions (social, physical, and economic) of the environment for health (see Box 1-2 for a list of the law's provisions of greatest relevance to public health and to this committee's work). Provisions pertaining to prevention and wellness offered in the act include the requirements for an absence of cost-sharing for recommended preventive services, for linking health-insurance premiums to participation in health-promotion programs, for public health workforce development (authorizes new training and placement programs for public health workers), and for community-based prevention activities. New community-based, prevention-focused grant programs have been created to target common *modifiable risk factors* rather than specific diseases. For example, community transformation grants will help local communities to address "policy, environmental, programmatic, and infrastructure changes needed to promote healthy living public access to key national indicators; develop a quality assurance framework to ensure rigorous and independent processes and quality data selection; and submit a report not later than 270 days after enactment of this Act, and annually thereafter, to the Commission outlining the findings and recommendations of the Academy).

(3) Creation of a Prevention and Wellness Trust Fund.[b]

(4) Expansion of the work of the Community Preventive Services Taskforce.

(5) Community Transformation grants.

(6) Funding for public health infrastructure and workforce (HHS, 2010a).[c]

---

[a] Established by executive order on June 10, 2010, to provide federal leadership by developing a national strategy with measurable goals (Executive Order No. 13544, 75 Fed. Reg. 33983 [June 10, 2010] http://edocket.access.gpo.gov/2010/pdf/2010-14613.pdf).

[b] The fund will provide $15 billion over 10 years. In FY 2010, the first $500 million of the Prevention and Public Health Fund was awarded: $250 million to bolster the primary-care workforce and $250 million for prevention and wellness activities broken down by category—$20 million to primary-care and behavioral-health integration, $70 million to public health infrastructure improvements for control of infectious disease and chronic disease, $21 million to fund information-gathering and aid strategic planning, $10 million to fund evidence-review task forces, and $23 million for public health workforce expansion and training (HHS, 2010a).

[c] For example, in September 2010, the Department of Health and Human Services awarded $16.8 million to train the public health workforce through support of 27 public health training centers in schools of public health and other public or nonprofit institutions from the Affordable Care Act Prevention and Public Health Fund (HHS, 2010b).

and reduce health disparities" (Public Law 111-148). The act also provides for community-based prevention activities through new regulatory and revenue authorities (for example, restaurant menu and vending-machine labeling requirements, mandatory break time for nursing mothers, and a 10 percent tax on indoor tanning services). In another provision of particular relevance to the present report (described more fully in Chapter 2), the act calls for a key national indicator system that will include health and is to be constructed with guidance from the National Academies.

CHARGE TO THE COMMITEEE

Recognizing the potential of systems-oriented public health approaches to achieve greater improvement in population health outcomes than changes in clinical care alone, the Robert Wood Johnson Foundation asked the Institute of Medicine (IOM) to convene a committee to review population health

---

BOX 1-3
Charge to the Committee on
Public Health Strategies to Improve Health

The committee will review population health strategies, associated metrics, and interventions in the context of a reformed health care system. The committee will review the role of score cards and other measures or assessments in summarizing the impact of the public health system, and how these can be used by policy-makers and the community to hold both government and other stakeholders accountable and to inform advocacy for public health policies and practices.

---

strategies, associated metrics, and interventions in the context of a reformed health care system. The Committee on Public Health Strategies to Improve Health was also asked (in the words of the charge given by the Robert Wood Johnson Foundation) to "review the role of score cards and other measures or assessments in summarizing the impact of the public health system, and how these can be used by policy-makers and the community to hold both government and other stakeholders accountable and to inform advocacy for public health policies and practices" (see Box 1-3).

The committee used two evidence-based notions as the starting point for its report. First, the committee believes that health strategies, interventions, and policies applied at the population level can advance current approaches to our nation's most pressing health concerns (such as obesity, infant mortality, injuries, cardiovascular disease, and health inequities) more efficiently and effectively than can isolated, intensive individual-level actions within the clinical care sector (see, for example, Woolf et al., 2007, estimating the effect on mortality of changes in one of the determinants of health, education). The Task Force on Community Preventive Services, which regularly reviews and evaluates research, has shown that strong evidence supports recommending some population-based interventions, such as reductions in blood alcohol concentration for their effectiveness in decreasing motor-vehicle injuries and deaths, and increases in prices of tobacco products for their effect on smoking initiation (Shults et al., 2001). The task force also recommends multicomponent interventions of several kinds: strong evidence was found to support mass-media campaigns in combination with other multisectoral strategies, including tobacco-price increases, school-based education, and other community education programs (Hopkins et al., 2001; Task Force on Community Preventive Services, 2001). The evidence base will grow as the task force's work expands with funding under the ACA and as the Cochrane Public Health Group (which published its first systematic review in February 2010, linking flexible work conditions with improved health) and other evidence-review bodies continue their work.

Second, the committee believes that measuring health outcomes and their determinants at both the individual level and the community level and in multiple sectors is an essential ingredient, with policy and resources, in motivating change, mobilizing action, measuring progress, and improving performance. As the clinical care community learned first, data can help to drive important improvements in performance (Berwick et al., 2003; Galvin and McGlynn, 2003). For the purposes of the more broadly conceived health system, data can also inform advocacy, public policy, and allocation of resources and can lead to better population health outcomes. High quality of data and measures is a prerequisite for good results—for example, how well does the evidence link indicators to the outcomes being measured (see, for example, Chassin et al., 2010)? The committee will address other "ingredients for change" in two future reports, on the law and on funding in the context of public health.

An important consideration in the ability to manage intersectoral collaboration among parts of the government and partnerships among government agencies and the private sector is the quality of governance—the ability to align potentially divergent interests toward a shared goal at local (city and county), state, and national levels. Because a public health agency is only one actor among many, there is increasing emphasis on engaging the highest-level elected officials, whether mayors, governors, or the president, to promote Health-in-All Policies—an approach that considers the implications on population health of policies in other sectors of government (e.g., transportation, land use, agriculture) and that uses such tools as health impact assessments, described elsewhere in this report (Kickbusch and Buckett, 2010; Stahl et al., 2006). The topic of governance is discussed briefly in Chapter 4 and will be addressed in more detail in the later report on the law and population health.

KEY TERMS

In its deliberations and in this report, the committee used the definition of the public health system provided in the 2003 IOM report *The Future of the Public's Health in the 21st Century*—an intersectoral, multistakeholder system whose core is the government public health infrastructure but also includes business, the clinical care delivery system, communities, schools, and nonprofit organizations (IOM, 2003). The 2003 figure (see Figure 1-1) did not explicitly refer to other components of government, but the current committee's report refers directly to the contributions of other government agencies or sectors that influence population health (such as those in trans-

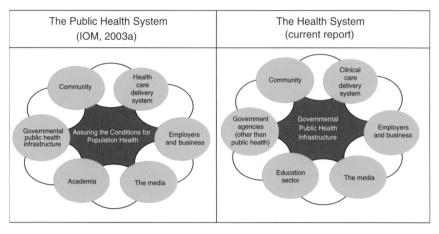

FIGURE 1-1 The health system.

NOTE: The present committee used the 2003 IOM committee's figure of the circle of system partners and description of the system (IOM, 2003) but renamed the system and made three revisions in the figure. They include placing the government public health infrastructure at the center, making it clear that other government agencies (non–public health agencies, including transportation, education, and others) are also key actors in the circle, and replacing health care with clinical care. The government public health agencies are in the center not because they are the most important in the population health system but because they are specifically tasked with ensuring the health of the public through their actions and by working with and through others. An additional change (Academia is now referred to as Education sector) acknowledges the considerable current and potential contributions of schools of all types to health.

portation, environment, economic development and land use planning, and education).

The overall public health system represented in Figure 1-1 is renamed simply *the health system,* with the health care delivery oval described more specifically as the *clinical care delivery system.* The modifiers *public* and *population* are poorly understood by persons other than public health professionals; use of them has made it both harder to understand that public health is about the population as a whole and easier to misinterpret or overlook the collective influence and responsibility that all sectors have for creating and sustaining the conditions necessary for health. In describing the system that comprises public health agencies, the clinical care delivery system, communities, and other partners as *the health system,* the committee seeks to reclaim the proper and evidence-based understanding of health not merely as clinical care but as the entirety of what we do as a society to create the conditions in which people can be healthy (IOM, 1988). The committee viewed as critical the need to focus policy-makers and the public on the complex interactions of multiple sectors that contribute to the production and maintenance of the health of Americans and the need to place contributions of the clinical care delivery system in perspective, including helping the public to understand the performance of the clinical care delivery system and its effects on population health.

In the present report, the committee uses the term *indicator* to refer to quantitative information that represents or is derived from statistics or measures (terms used interchangeably in the statistics community) that are developed by federal statistical agencies and other producers of data. Indicators are designed to be communicated to policy-makers or to the public. They may be simple (such as a disease-specific death rate in a particular age group) or complex (such as a composite figure that incorporates several types of data, for example, the Human Development Index[4]). Indicators are available for most steps in the process to health improvement—that is, indicators of resources; of capacities; of interventions, processes, and policies; of health outcomes; and performance. The term *information* is used, as in the 2003 IOM report, to refer generally to three distinct terms in information science: data, information (data put into context through analysis), and knowledge (Lumpkin, 2001).

TWO PARADIGMS

The committee contrasted two health paradigms and two corresponding approaches: the biomedical (or clinical) paradigm and the broader ecologic (or determinants-of-health) paradigm. Into the early part of the 20th century, changes in the means of production and in sanitation led to vast decreases in infectious disease and improvements in quality of life. In the latter half of the 20th century, biomedical science and greater understanding of the biologic basis of disease strongly shaped expert and popular understanding of the causes of poor health (CDC, 1999). The results were a proliferation of diagnostic and therapeutic technologies designed for individuals and, in time, the emergence of the biomedical model as the dominant paradigm for viewing health and its improvement (Fielding et al., 2010). The biomedical model is also associated with the emergence of insurance mechanisms to pay for new technologies and interventions and with the large increases in costs. The two paradigms are complementary, and a balanced investment in both would create health policy that produces improved health.

The World Health Organization has defined health as "a state of physical, mental and social well-being and not merely the absence of dis-

---

[4] See, for example, Social Science Research Council (2009).

ease or infirmity" (WHO, 1948).[5] Public health has been defined as "what we, as a society, do collectively to assure the conditions for people to be healthy" (IOM, 1988, 2003). The ecologic (or determinants-of-health and population-based) health model encompasses but is much broader than the clinical model, which is focused on pathophysiologic causes of individual risk factors for disease and injury. The perspective that informs the ecologic model is rooted in an examination of the "relationship between the innate biologic characteristics of individuals and their interactions with their peer groups, families, communities, schools and workplaces, as well as the broad economic, cultural, social, and physical environmental conditions at the local, national, and global levels" (Fielding et al., 2010, p. 176).

The committee reiterates an illustration of the determinants of health provided in the 2003 IOM report *The Future of the Public's Health in the 21st Century* (IOM, 2003; see Figure 1-2). The clinical care model focuses largely on the two innermost circles (individual genes and biology, features of a disease, and behavior). In contrast with the highly specialized and individualized approaches of clinical medicine, health-improvement strategies that stem from the ecologic model are developed to address social and physical environments that influence patterns of disease and injury and human responses to them over the life cycle (Kindig and Stoddart, 2003). Interventions reflecting the latter (ecologic) model—from policies on air quality and living wages to health-promotion programs that target nutrition and physical activity—may have wide-ranging effects on multiple disease states (see Table 2-1 for examples). A healthy community has been described in various ways: for example, one where all sectors contribute to create social and physical environments that foster health. In practice, such a community meets basic needs: access to affordable, healthy foods; affordable housing and transportation; and such essential services as medical care and education. It offers a sustainable, healthful environment with clean air and water, open space and parks, low levels of toxic exposures and low emissions, and affordable, sustainable energy (Fielding et al., 2010). The present report argues that data can help communities to assess their status in those respects and to take steps to improve conditions for health with the ultimate goal of improving population health outcomes.

Human behavior of individuals (the second circle from the center in Figure 1-2) is strongly conditioned by people's social frame of reference and relationships; such social institutions as school, religious congregations, and workplaces; income and economic conditions; and physical environments (see, for example, Evans et al., 1990). It is also influenced by

---

[5] Preamble to the Constitution of the World Health Organization as adopted by the International Health Conference, New York, 19–22 June 1946; signed on 22 July 1946 by the representatives of 61 States (Official Records of the World Health Organization, no. 2, p. 100) and entered into force on 7 April 1948 (WHO, 1948).

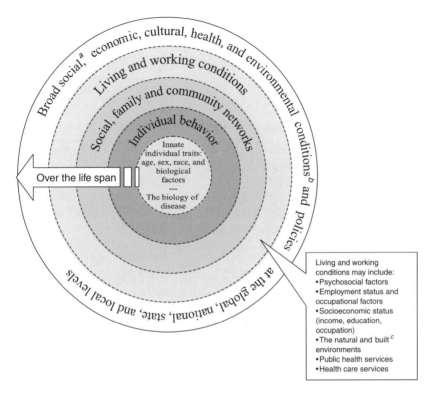

FIGURE 1-2 A guide to thinking about the determinants of population health.

ª Social conditions include economic inequality, urbanization, mobility, cultural values, and attitudes and policies related to discrimination and intolerance on the basis of race, sex, and other differences.

ᵇ Other conditions at [the] national level might include major sociopolitical shifts, such as recession, war, and government collapse. The built environment includes transportation, water and sanitation, housing, and other dimensions under [the] auspices of urban planning.

ᶜ The built environment includes transportation, water and sanitation, housing, and other dimensions of urban planning.

SOURCE: Adapted from Dahlgren and Whitehead (1991). Dotted lines between levels of model denote interaction effects between and among various levels of health determinants (Worthman, 1999).

genetic constitution (the innermost circle), whose expression is in turn affected by interactions with environmental conditions. Inputs from multiple sectors correspond to determinants of health in diverse ways. For example, the social environment—which includes social capital, safety, and school policies—can be addressed through interventions for access to healthy food, agricultural policy, cultural programming, and physical activities. Economic determinants, such as income and employment, can be addressed through living-wage policies, unemployment support, and retraining. Measures of those domains may assess social well-being or fresh-food availability, policy effectiveness, and program use.

The Evidence on Determinants of Health

Recognition of the determinants of health is well documented, but several milestones warrant highlighting, including Geoffrey Rose's *Strategy of Preventive Medicine* (1992), which examined patterns of disease in populations; Evans and Stoddart's article "Producing Health, Consuming Health Care" (1990); and the 2008 report of the World Health Organization Commission on Social Determinants of Health, *Closing the Gap in a Generation: Health Equity Through Action on the Social Determinants of Health* (Commission on Social Determinants of Health, 2008).

A robust and expanding peer-reviewed literature addresses the associations between the upstream determinants of health—social, economic, and environmental—and poor health outcomes and between socioeconomic inequality and poor health. Researchers have found that poverty, low levels of education, lower social status, and income inequality are linked with higher mortality and higher rates of poor health, with more or stronger evidence regarding some conditions (see, for example, Berkman and Kawachi, 2000; Carstairs and Morris, 1989; Daniels et al., 2000; Kaplan, 1996; Kennedy et al., 1998; Kogevinas et al., 1991; Marmot and Wilkinson, 1999). The Whitehall I and II studies of British civil servants, which controlled for an array of variables but still found a steep difference in mortality between the highest and lowest grades of civil-service employment, remain classics of the literature on determinants of health (Marmot et al., 1991). Neighborhood conditions (including deprivation, poor housing, violence, and other stressors) are also associated with worse health status (Ellen et al., 2001; Kawachi and Berkman, 2003; Yen and Kaplan, 1999).

Epidemiologists studying the relationships between health and the social environment generally describe three dimensions: the role of socioeconomics (for example, income, employment, and education); the role of social structure (for example, social institutions and phenomena, including discrimination and income inequality); and the quality of the social, built, and natural environment (for example, social cohesion, social capital, and civic engagement). The peer-reviewed literature contains evidence on the social environment and its relationship to asthma (Cagney and Browning, 2004; Williams et al., 2009; Wright, 2006) and to health risk behaviors, such as smoking (Kleinschmidt et al., 1995; Shohaimi et al., 2003); evidence on its relationship to birth weight shows the transgenerational effect of neighborhood poverty during pregnancy (Collins et al., 2003, 2009; O'Campo et al., 1997; Schempf et al., 2009). And an increasing body of evidence sheds light on the relationship between access to healthy food and obesity (California Center for Public Health Advocacy et al., 2008; Larson et al., 2009; Morland et al., 2006). The mechanisms by which socioeconomic conditions can influence health outcomes, such as asthma, include chronic exposure to social stressors that can lead to changes in the brain and the immune system (Lantz and Pritchard, 2010).

The built environment (land use patterns, the transportation system, and design features) has seen increased research attention in recent years. Although there are still gaps in the evidence base and conceptual complexities (given the many mediators at work, including social and cultural variables and such psychosocial factors as feelings of safety and security), the influence of the built environment in constraining or facilitating physical activity is increasingly clear (TRB and IOM, 2005).

The Evidence on Interventions to Address Determinants of Health

Altering root causes (the determinants of health) to create healthy communities is challenging because they form or are woven into the very fabric of family, community, and societal structures. Strong, supportive families and communities foster safe, secure environments and build social capital. Public-sector and private-sector structures and systems, through policies and norms, provide social infrastructure and shape lives. Linear[6] approaches involving one or two sectors to solve such complex health challenges will necessarily be modest in effect (Leischow and Milstein, 2006). Broad action on multiple determinants involving multiple sectors is needed to achieve greater effects on population health.

Unlike clinical interventions that focus on downstream factors (for example, individual-level factors), such as using prescription medication to lower blood sugar concentrations or blood pressure, population health interventions by public health agencies and their partners can address a broader spectrum of causation ranging from proximal conditions that lead to unhealthy behaviors and exposures in communities to sick people's need for services in the medical care delivery system. Upstream strategies (aiming to affect root causes or underlying issues before they lead to poor individual health outcomes downstream) include policies and interventions that affect the social and physical environments, as illustrated in Table 2-1. These strategies demonstrate the versatility of population health interventions in reducing the burden of illness and injury and in advancing wellness by altering conditions that affect what people eat, drink, breathe, inhabit, work and

---

[6] That is, assuming simple cause–effect relationships.

play with, and use (CDC, 1999; Frieden, 2010). There is also evidence that interventions in two components of the built environment—land use (for example, accessibility of public recreational venues) and transportation— can affect community health (Bauman and Bull, 2007; Davison and Lawson, 2006; Ewing et al., 2002; Handy et al., 2002) in areas that relate to physical activity, healthy eating, and obesity (Brownson et al., 2006).

Bold changes in clean air laws and tobacco taxes helped to transform social norms and led to reductions in cigarette-smoking. Box 1-4 shows how interventions at the population level can offer greater returns on investment than can clinical care alone.

Evidence on the effectiveness of interventions is more substantive when one considers the intermediate determinants and outcomes, such as behaviors that are risk factors for chronic disease (as described above). As one moves further upstream, to the outermost ring of the illustration in Figure 1-2, although strong evidence links health outcomes to various dimensions of the socioeconomic environment (such as education, income, housing and neighborhood quality, social cohesion, and social capital) and suggests some potential loci for interventions, there is still a dearth of evidence on the most effective interventions on many topics (see Bambra et al.,

---

BOX 1-4
Value of Population-Level Interventions

Interventions at the population level (such as smoking laws, school programs, and motor-vehicle safety laws) can have greater cost savings than those at the individual level. For example, medical care accounts for the largest proportion of the direct costs of smoking. "Men who smoke incur $15,800 (in 2002 dollars) more in lifetime medical expenses than non-smokers, and women who smoke incur $17,500 more than non-smokers." In 1999, the state [CA] "spent $8,564,623 in total health care costs directly attributable to smoking, including $4,016,568 in hospital care, $2,060,234 in outpatient care, and $1,133,432 for prescriptions" (California Benefits Review Program, 2006).

A 2009 RAND study shows that reducing Americans' average intake of sodium to the amount recommended by health officials could save the nation billions of dollars annually in avoided medical care costs and improve the quality of life of millions of people (RAND, 2009). The study estimates that meeting national sodium guidelines could eliminate 11 million cases of high blood pressure nationally. In just one calendar year, that would save 312,000 quality-adjusted life years with a monetary value of an estimated $32 billion (Palar and Sturm, 2009). Population-based strategies (such as redesigning food-labeling information and manufacturers' voluntarily lowering of sodium concentrations in their products) would have multiple health effects (such as avoiding hypertension and the resulting cardiovascular disease and treatment) (Bibbins-Domingo et al., 2010).

2010). Several examples—the US Head Start Program (Administration for Children and Families, 2010) and other early child-development programs, such as the Nurse-Family Partnership (Olds, 2002; Olds et al., 2007), or early academic-enrichment programs (Reynolds et al., 2007)—suggest that addressing the more upstream determinants of health can be effective. The remaining conceptual and methodologic challenges and gaps include defining socioeconomic environments and elucidating the complex and interrelated pathways between many determinants and health outcomes of interest. For example, higher levels of educational attainment are strongly linked with better health outcomes, but there are multiple confounding influences, including neighborhood conditions, early life experiences, and race and ethnicity (Woolf et al., 2007). And there are challenges in linking specific determinants of health to specific outcomes and, in cases in which the evidence of an association is strong, in establishing what interventions are most effective in addressing the determinants of health.

A primary challenge in research on population-based interventions is that the traditional gold standard technique of randomized controlled trials is not always feasible or appropriate in the public health context (for example, given the complexity of causal factors and the levels on which interventions function). However, other statistical techniques (such as observational studies and quasi-experimental study designs) may be used (Rosenbaum, 2002, 2010), as may tools offered by other disciplines (such as economics and the social sciences), to demonstrate the effectiveness of public health approaches. Such tools as health impact assessments can lead to syntheses of the best available evidence, and predictive modeling can supplement the evidence base (see, for example, Thomson et al., 2008). An additional contributor to the dearth of evidence about what works to address specific determinants of health are deficiencies in the reporting of public health intervention research (Armstrong et al., 2008).

MEETING THE CHARGE

To meet its charge, the committee reflected on the implications of the Affordable Care Act and the case for moving toward a population health approach as seen through the lens of measurement of health outcomes and system performance. The committee held three information-gathering meetings on public health measurement and reviewed the relevant literature (peer-reviewed journals and reports and white papers). Each meeting involved an array of stakeholders (see the agendas in Appendix C). After each information-gathering meeting, the committee met in closed session (and held two additional meetings that were closed to the public) to allow committee deliberation and discussion. In this report's remaining three chapters (and seven recommendations), the committee discusses measurement-based system improvements to support all partners in the health system, from the public health agencies and their clinical care counterparts to various community and private-sector organizations, in becoming more knowledgeable about population health outcomes and their determinants and in developing, implementing, and evaluating programs, policies, and interventions to improve health.

WHAT THIS REPORT DOES *NOT* ADDRESS

As discussed in this chapter and throughout the report, a population's health is influenced by a multitude of factors that overlap and span many disciplines and topics. The committee aims to cover many of the topics through its three reports—the present one and two later ones. Each is intended to view population health improvement through a different lens (measurement, the law, and funding). The preface of this report describes the areas of overlap among the three overarching topics and explains that although each has unique characteristics and effects on health, none can be looked at exclusively without discussing the others. In the present report, on measurement and health, the committee uses the scope of measurement as a tool to improve population health. This report focuses on measurement and on the US population health statistics and information system (which collects, analyzes, and reports population health data, clinical care data, and health-relevant information from other sectors). However, it is important to note that the committee did not attempt to prepare a comprehensive and systematic catalog or evaluation of all activities (national, state, and local) to put forth health indicators or indicators of well-being. The committee referred to two overviews of indicator efforts in the health field (Public Health Institute, 2010; Wold, 2008) and a more general summary of key indicators (on multiple topics beyond health, including the economy, society, and the environment) contained in the Government Accountability Office's report *Informing Our Nation: Improving How to Understand and Assess the USA's Position and Progress* (GAO, 2004).

This IOM report notes topics for later reports of the committee, but it does not examine them in any depth. For example, many of the committee's recommendations (in Chapters 3 and 4) call for increases or changes in resources, staffing, or allocations of funds. Other subjects related to measurement that the committee will review in more detail in its later reports on the law and funding include

- accountability,
- governance (and governing bodies),
- innovative ways to use the law on the basis of what is learned though measurement,

- inadequacy of resources available to government statistical agencies,
- allocation of funding for public health agencies,
- the mismatch between the targets of public health funding and the leading causes of preventable deaths and illnesses,
- the public health role in monitoring clinical care quality and outcomes through the use of personal health information, and
- the effects of health care reform on the structure of public health agencies.

The committee continues to hold information-gathering meetings and to research public health law and funding, and the issues noted above and other issues identified during that process will be raised in its two forthcoming reports.

REFERENCES

Administration for Children and Families. 2010. *About the Office of Head Start*. http://www. acf.hhs.gov/programs/ohs/about/index.html#factsheet (November 3, 2010).

Armstrong, R., E. Waters, L. Moore, E. Riggs, L. G. Cuervo, P. Lumbiganon, and P. Hawe. 2008. Improving the reporting of public health intervention research: Advancing trend and consort. *Journal of Public Health* 30(1):103-109.

Bambra, C., M. Gibson, A. Sowden, K. Wright, M. Whitehead, and M. Petticrew. 2010. Tackling the wider social determinants of health and health inequalities: Evidence from systematic reviews. *Journal of Epidemiology and Community Health* 64(4):284-291.

Bauman, A. E., and F. C. Bull. 2007. *Environmental Correlates of Physical Activity and Walking in Adults and Children*. London, England: National Institute of Health and Clinical Excellence.

Berkman, L. F., and I. Kawachi, eds. 2000. *Social Epidemiology*. New York: Oxford University Press.

Berwick, D. M., N. A. DeParle, D. M. Eddy, P. M. Ellwood, A. C. Enthoven, G. C. Halvorson, K. W. Kizer, E. A. McGlynn, U. E. Reinhardt, R. D. Reischauer, W. L. Roper, J. W. Rowe, L. D. Schaeffer, J. E. Wennberg, and G. R. Wilensky. 2003. Paying for performance: Medicare should lead. *Health Affairs* 22(6):8-10.

Bibbins-Domingo, K., G. M. Chertow, P. G. Coxson, A. Moran, J. M. Lightwood, M. J. Pletcher, and L. Goldman. 2010. Projected effect of dietary salt reductions on future cardiovascular disease. *New England Journal of Medicine* 362:590-599.

Booske, B. C., J. K. Athens, D. A. Kindig, H. Park, and P. L. Remington. 2009. *Different Perspectives for Assigning Weights to Determinants of Health: County Health Rankings Working Paper*. Madison: University of Wisconsin Population Health Institute.

Brownson, R. C., D. Haire-Joshu, and D. A. Luke. 2006. Shaping the context of health: A review of environmental and policy approaches in the prevention of chronic diseases. *Annual Review of Public Health* 27(1):341-370.

Cagney, K. A., and C. R. Browning. 2004. Exploring neighborhood-level variation in asthma and other respiratory diseases—the contribution of neighborhood social context. *Journal of General Internal Medicine* 19(3):229-236.

California Benefits Review Program. 2006. *Criteria and Guidelines for the Analysis of Long-Term Impacts on Healthcare Costs and Public Health: California Health Benefits Review Program*. Oakland, CA: University of California, Office of the President.

California Center for Public Health Advocacy, PolicyLink, and UCLA Center for Health Policy Research. 2008. *Designed for Disease: The Link Between Local Food Environments and Obesity and Diabetes.* Los Angeles, CA: UCLA Center for Health Policy Research.

Carstairs, V., and R. Morris. 1989. Deprivation and health. *British Medical Journal* 299(6713): 1462-1462.

CDC (Centers for Disease Control and Prevention). 1999. *Ten Great Public Health Achievements—United States, 1900-1999.* http://www.cdc.gov/mmwr/preview/mmwr html/00056796.htm (September 8, 2010).

Chassin, M. R., J. Loeb, and S. P. Schmaltz. 2010. Accountability measures—using measurement to promote quality improvement. *New England Journal of Medicine* 363:683-688.

Collins, J. W., Jr., R. J. David, N. G. Prachand, and M. L. Pierce. 2003. Low birth weight across generations. *Maternal and Child Health Journal* 7(4):229-237.

Collins, J. W., Jr., J. Wambach, R. J. David, and K. M. Rankin. 2009. Women's lifelong exposure to neighborhood poverty and low birth weight: A population-based study. *Maternal and Child Health Journal* 13(3):326-333.

Commission on Social Determinants of Health. 2008. *Closing the Gap in a Generation.* Geneva, Switzerland: World Health Organization.

Commonwealth Fund. 2009. *The Path to a High Performance US Health System: A 2020 vision and the policies to pave the way.* New York: Commonwealth Fund.

Cutler, D. M., A. B. Rosen, and S. Vijan. 2006. The value of medical spending in the United States, 1960–2000. *New England Journal of Medicine* 355(9):920-927.

Dahlgren, G., and M. Whitehead. 1991. *Policies and strategies to promote social equity in health.* Stockholm, Sweden: Institute for Future Studies.

Daniels, M. J., F. Dominici, J. M. Samet, and S. L. Zeger. 2000. Estimating particulate matter-mortality dose-response curves and threshold levels: An analysis of daily time-series for the 20 largest U.S. cities. *American Journal of Epidemiology* 152(5):397-406.

Davis, K., C. Schoen, K. Shea, and C. Haran. 2008. Aiming high for the U.S. health system: A context for health reform. *The Journal of Law, Medicine & Ethics* 36(4):629-643.

Davis, K., C. Schoen, and K. Stremikis. 2010. *Mirror, Mirror on the Wall: How the Performance of the U.S. Health Care System Compares Internationally—2010 update.* Washington, DC: Commonwealth Fund.

Davison, K., and C. Lawson. 2006. Do attributes in the physical environment influence children's physical activity? A review of the literature. *International Journal of Behavioral Nutrition and Physical Activity* 3(1):19.

Doty, M. M., and A. L. Holmgren. 2006. *HealthCare Disconnect: Gaps in Coverage and Care for Minority Adults. Findings from the Commonwealth Fund Biennial Health Insurance Survey (2005).* New York: The Commonwealth Fund.

Ellen, I. G., T. Mijanovich, and K. N. Dillman. 2001. Neighborhood effects on health: Exploring the links and assessing the evidence. *Journal of Urban Affairs* 23(3-4):391-408.

Evans, R. G., M. L. Barer, and T. R. Marmor, eds. 1990. *Why are Some People Healthy and Others Not?: The Determinants of Health of Populations.* New York: Walter de Gruyter.

Evans, R. G., and G. L. Stoddart. 1990. Producing health, consuming health-care. *Social Science & Medicine* 31(12):1347-1363.

Ewing, R., R. Pendall, and D. Chen. 2002. *Measuring Sprawl and its Impact: Volume 1.* Washington, DC: Smart Growth America.

Executive Office of the President, Council of Economic Advisers. 2009. *The Economic Case for Health Care Reform.* Washington, DC: Government Printing Office.

Fielding, J. E., S. M. Teutch, and L. Breslow. 2010. A framework for public health in the United States. *Public Health Reviews* 32(1):174-189.

Frieden, T. R. 2010. A framework for public health action: The health impact pyramid. *American Journal of Public Health* 100(4):590-595.

Galvin, R. S., and E. A. McGlynn. 2003. Using performance measurement to drive improvement—a road map for change. *Medical Care* 41(1):I48-I60.

GAO (Government Accountability Office). 2004. *Informing Our Nation: Improving How to Understand and Assess the USA's Position and Progress—Report to the Chairman, Subcommittee on Science, Technology, and Space, Committee on Commerce, Science, and Transportation, U.S. Senate.* Washington, DC: GAO.

Handy, S. L., M. G. Boarnet, R. Ewing, and R. E. Killingsworth. 2002. How the built environment affects physical activity: Views from urban planning. *American Journal of Preventive Medicine* 23(2S):64-73.

HealthCare.gov. 2010. *Understanding the Affordable Care Act: Introduction.* http://www.healthcare.gov/law/introduction (November 12, 2010).

Hewitt Associates. 2009. *Health Care Reform: The Perils of Inaction and the Promise of Effective Action.* Lincolnshire, IL: Hewitt Associates.

HHS (Department of Health and Human Services). 2010a. *Affordable Care Act: Laying the Foundation for Prevention.* http://www.healthreform.gov/about/index.html (June 22, 2010).

HHS. 2010b. *HHS Awards $16.8 Million to Train Public Health Workforce: Grants Awarded to 27 Public Health Training Centers.* http://www.hhs.gov/news/press/2010 pres/09/20100913a.html (November 12, 2010).

HHS, Public Health Services, and CDC. 1994. *For the Health of a Nation: Returns on Investment in Public Health.* Washington, DC: HHS.

Hopkins, D. P., P. A. Briss, C. J. Ricard, C. G. Husten, V. G. Carande-Kulis, J. E. Fielding, M. O. Alao, J. W. McKenna, D. J. Sharp, J. R. Harris, T. A. Woollery, and K. W. Harris. 2001. Reviews of evidence regarding interventions to reduce tobacco use and exposure to environmental tobacco smoke. *American Journal of Preventive Medicine* 20(2, Suppl 1):16-66.

IOM (Institute of Medicine). 1988. *The Future of Public Health.* Washington, DC: National Academy Press.

IOM. 2003. *The Future of the Public's Health in the 21st Century.* Washington, DC: The National Academies Press.

Kaiser Family Foundation and Health Research and Educational Trust. 2007. *Employer Health Benefits 2007 Annual Survey.* Menlo Park, CA: Kaiser Family Foundation and Health Research and Educational Trust.

Kaiser Family Foundation and Health Research and Educational Trust. 2009. *Employer Health Benefits: 2009 Annual Survey.* Menlo Park, CA: Kaiser Family Foundation and Health Research and Educational Trust.

Kaplan, G. A. 1996. People and places: Contrasting perspectives on the association between social class and health. *International Journal of Health Services* 26(3):507-519.

Kawachi, I., and L. F. Berkman, eds. 2003. *Neighborhoods and Health.* New York: Oxford University Press.

Kennedy, B. P., I. Kawachi, D. Prothrow-Stith, K. Lochner, and V. Gupta. 1998. Social capital, income inequality, and firearm violent crime. *Social Science & Medicine* 47(1):7-17.

Kickbusch, I., and K. Buckett. 2010. *Implementing Health in All Policies: Adelaide 2010.* Adelaide, South Australia: Department of Health, Government of South Australia.

Kindig, D., and G. Stoddart. 2003. What is population health? *American Journal of Public Health* 93(3):380-383.

Kleinschmidt, I., M. Hills, and P. Elliott. 1995. Smoking behaviour can be predicted by neighbourhood deprivation measures. *Journal of Epidemiology and Community Health* 49(Suppl 2):S72-S77.

Kogevinas, M., M. G. Marmot, and A. J. Fox. 1991. Socioeconomic differences in cancer survival. *Journal of Epidemiology and Community Health* 45:216-219.

Lantz, P. M., and A. Pritchard. 2010. Socioeconomic indicators that matter for population health. *Preventing Chronic Disease Public Health Research, Practice and Policy* 7(4). http://www.cdc.gov/pcd/issues/2010/jul/09_0246.htm (July 9, 2010).

Larson, N. I., M. T. Story, and M. C. Nelson. 2009. Neighborhood environments: Disparities in access to healthy foods in the U.S. *American Journal of Preventive Medicine* 36(1):74-81.

Leischow, S. J., and B. Milstein. 2006. Systems thinking and modeling for public health practice. *American Journal of Public Health* 96(3):403-405.

Lumpkin, J. R. 2001. Air, water, places, and data—public health in the information age. *Journal of Public Health Management & Practice* 7(6):22-30.

Marmot, M., and R. G. Wilkinson, eds. 1999. *Social Determinants of Health*. New York: Oxford Press.

Marmot, M. G., S. Stansfeld, C. Patel, F. North, J. Head, I. White, E. Brunner, A. Feeney, and G. D. Smith. 1991. Health inequalities among british civil servants: The Whitehall II study. *The Lancet* 337(8754):1387-1393.

McGinnis, J. M., and W. H. Foege. 1993. Actual causes of death in the United States. *Journal of the American Medical Association* 270(18):2007-2012.

McGinnis, J. M., P. Williams-Russo, and J. R. Knickman. 2002. The case for more active policy attention to health promotion. *Health Affairs* 21(2):78-93.

Morland, K., A. V. Diez Roux, and S. Wing. 2006. Supermarkets, other food stores, and obesity: The atherosclerosis risk in communities study. *American Journal of Preventive Medicine* 30(4):333-339.

National Prevention Health Promotion and Public Health Council. 2010. *2010 Annual Status Report*. Washington, DC: HHS.

Nolte, E., and C. M. McKee. 2008. Measuring the health of nations: Updating an earlier analysis. *Health Affairs* 27(1):58-71.

O'Campo, P., X. Xue, M. C. Wang, and M. Caughy. 1997. Neighborhood risk factors for low birth weight in Baltimore: A multilevel analysis. *American Journal of Public Health* 87(7):1113-1118.

OECD (Organisation for Economic Co-operation and Development). 2009. *OECD Health Data 2009: Statistics and Indicators for 30 Countries*. Paris, France: OECD.

Olds, D. L. 2002. Prenatal and infancy home visiting by nurses: From randomized trials to community replication. *Prevention Science* 3(3):153-172.

Olds, D. L., H. Kitzman, C. Hanks, R. Cole, E. Anson, K. Sidora-Arcoleo, D. W. Luckey, C. R. Henderson, Jr., J. Holmberg, R. A. Tutt, A. J. Stevenson, and J. Bondy. 2007. Effects of nurse home visiting on maternal and child functioning: Age-9 follow-up of a randomized trial. *Pediatrics* 120(4):e832-e845.

Palar, K., and R. Sturm. 2009. Potential societal savings from reduced sodium consumption in the US adult population. *American Journal of Health Promotion* 24(1):49-57.

Public Health Institute. 2010. *Data Sets, Data Platforms, Data Utility: Resource Compendium*. Oakland, CA: Public Health Institute.

RAND. 2009. *Lowering Sodium Consumption Could Save US $18 Billion Annually in Health Costs*. Santa Monica, CA: RAND Corporation.

Reynolds, A. J., J. A. Temple, S.-R. Ou, D. L. Robertson, J. P. Mersky, J. W. Topitzes, and M. D. Niles. 2007. Effects of a school-based, early childhood intervention on adult health and well-being: A 19-year follow-up of low-income families. *Archives of Pediatrics and Adolescent Medicine* 161(8):730-739.

Rose, G. 1992. *The Strategy of Preventive Medicine*. New York: Oxford University Press.

Rosenbaum, P. R. 2002. *Observational Studies*. 2nd ed., *Springer Series in Statistics*. New York: Springer.

Rosenbaum, P. R. 2010. A matched observational study. In *Design of Observational Studies*, Springer series in statistics. New York: Springer. Pp. 153-161.

Schempf, A., D. Strobino, and P. O'Campo. 2009. Neighborhood effects on birthweight: An exploration of psychosocial and behavioral pathways in Baltimore, 1995-1996. *Social Science & Medicine* 68(1):100-110.

Schoen, C., S. R. Collins, J. L. Kriss, and M. M. Doty. 2008. How many are underinsured? Trends among U.S. Adults, 2003 and 2007. *Health Affairs* 27(4):w298-w309.

Shohaimi, S., R. Luben, N. Wareham, N. Day, S. Bingham, A. Welch, S. Oakes, and K. T. Khaw. 2003. Residential area deprivation predicts smoking habit independently of individual educational level and occupational social class. A cross sectional study in the norfolk cohort of the european investigation into cancer (EPIC-Norfolk). *Journal of Epidemiology and Community Health* 57(4):270-276.

Shults, R. A., R. W. Elder, D. A. Sleet, J. L. Nichols, M. O. Alao, V. G. Carande-Kulis, S. Zaza, D. M. Sosin, and R. S. Thompson. 2001. Reviews of evidence regarding interventions to reduce alcohol-impaired driving. *American Journal of Preventive Medicine* 21(4, Suppl 1):66-88.

Social Science Research Council. 2009. *Methodology: The American Human Development Index*. Brooklyn, NY: Social Science Research Council.

Stahl, T., M. Wismar, E. Ollila, E. Lahtinen, and K. Leppo, eds. 2006. *Health in All Policies, Prospects and Potentials*. Finland: Finnish Ministry of Social Affairs and Health.

Task Force on Community Preventive Services. 2001. Recommendations regarding interventions to reduce tobacco use and exposure to environmental tobacco smoke. *American Journal of Preventive Medicine* 20(2S):10-15.

Thomson, H., R. Jepson, F. Hurley, and M. Douglas. 2008. Assessing the unintended health impacts of road transport policies and interventions: Translating research evidence for use in policy and practice. *Biomedical Central Public Health* 8:339.

TRB (Transportation Research Board), and IOM. 2005. *Does the Built Environment Influence Physical Activity? Examining the Evidence: Special Report 282*. Washington, DC: National Academies Press.

Truffer, C. J., S. Keehan, S. Smith, J. Cylus, A. Sisko, and J. A. Poisal. 2010. Health spending projections through 2019. The recession's impact continues. *Health Affairs* 29(3):522-529.

WHO (World Health Organization). 1948. *WHO definition of health*. http://www.who.int/about/definition/en/print.html (September 8, 2010).

Williams, D. R., M. Sternthal, and R. J. Wright. 2009. Social determinants: Taking the social context of asthma seriously. *Pediatrics* 123 (Suppl 3):S174-184.

Wold, C. 2008. *Health Indicators: A Review of Reports Currently in Use*. Conducted for The State of the USA. Wold and Associates.

Woolf, S. H., R. E. Johnson, R. L. Phillips, Jr., and M. Philipsen. 2007. Giving everyone the health of the educated: An examination of whether social change would save more lives than medical advances. *American Journal of Public Health* 97(4):679-683.

Woolf, S. H., R. M. Jones, R. E. Johnson, R. L. Phillips, Jr., M. N. Oliver, A. Bazemore, and A. Vichare. 2010. Avertable deaths associated with household income in Virginia. *American Journal of Public Health* 100(4):750-755.

Worthman, C. M. 1999. Epidemiology of human development. In *Hormones, Health, and Behaviors: A Socio-Ecological and Lifespan Perspective*, edited by C. Panter-Brick and C. M. Worthman. Cambridge: Cambridge University Press. Pp. 47-104.

Wright, R. J. 2006. Health effects of socially toxic neighborhoods: The violence and urban asthma paradigm. *Clinics in Chest Medicine* 27(3):413-421.

Yen, I. H., and G. A. Kaplan. 1999. Poverty area residence and changes in depression and perceived health status: Evidence from the Alameda County study. *International Journal of Epidemiology* 28(1):90-94.

2

Needed: An Information Enterprise to Drive Knowledge and Population Health Improvement

The national preoccupation with the cost of clinical care is well founded, and changes in the system are essential and urgent. However, improving the clinical care delivery system's efficiency and effectiveness is likely to have only a narrow effect on the overall health of the population. Other factors, or determinants of health—genes, behaviors, social and economic conditions, and environmental exposures—influence health outcomes. The national emphasis on clinical care (largely to the exclusion of other contributors to health) has not led to health outcomes that are commensurate with investments. A landmark 1974 Canadian government report provided one of the earliest acknowledgments that clinical care alone is neither responsible for poor health outcomes nor the sole solution to health problems (Lalonde, 1981). In the ensuing decades, the evidence supporting that thesis has grown (see Chapter 1 for further discussion).

In the present chapter, the committee discusses the information needs of the health system (broadly conceived) and the capacities and limitations of the nation's population health statistics and information system, which consists of an array of public-sector and private-sector entities that collect, analyze, and study data and communicate information relevant to population health. The system's familiar components include vital-records systems; surveillance systems (for example, for acute conditions); and such clinical care data sources as administrative claims databases, electronic health records, and federal surveys that summarize population health outcomes (NCVHS, 2010).[1]

Helping communities to understand the local conditions for health and outcomes is a necessary (but not sufficient) precursor of the work of improving unfavorable socioeconomic and physical environments. Accurate, timely, locally relevant information is crucial for the implementation of population-focused interventions of established effectiveness and for implementing and evaluating promising new strategies. In the pages that follow, the committee discusses three sets of challenges, endeavors in which changes are warranted to strengthen the population health statistics and information system: adopting the determinants-of-health perspective at a fundamental level (to complement the health system's predominantly biomedical orientation); enhancing responsiveness to the needs of end users; and coordination and cross-sector collaboration at the national level, beginning with the primary federal health-statistics agency—the National Center for Health Statistics (NCHS)—and with federal health data and statistics activities in general.[2] An additional, overarching challenge, and one to which the committee intends to return in its later report on funding, is the extreme inadequacy of resources available for statistical and data-gathering activities of governmental public health agencies at all levels in general (Friedman and Parrish, 2009b; HHS et al., 2002) and NCHS in particular (NCHS, 2008, 2009; Population Association of America, 2010).

Several related terms are used to describe concepts in the field of health statistics and information. In common professional usage, the terms *statistics* and *measures* are often used interchangeably to refer to an aggregate data point (or set of data points) about a phenomenon, such as disease-specific mortality in a particular age group over a given period. (Statistic is also used in the field to indicate a type of measure, such as a mean, a median, or a proportion.) A specific statistic or measure is commonly called an indicator when it is widely acknowledged to be useful for monitoring something of concern to policy-makers or to the public. Examples include the monthly unemployment rate and the annual poverty rate as indicators of the health of the national economy. Such indicators can be simple statistics or can be quite complex; for example, many data sources go into the

---

[1] The system includes 57 vital registration jurisdictions in the United States and the entities represented by the National Association for Public Health Statistics and Information Systems (Schwartz, 2008).

[2] The Department of Health and Human Services (HHS) Data Council plays a key role in facilitating intradepartment coordination on data and statistics issues. The council has supported the development of the HHS Gateway to Data and Statistics (HHS, 2010d), which represents one of several HHS efforts to make federal health data more available and accessible. The council's role in coordinating HHS data systems has also been discussed in a meeting of the HHS secretary's Advisory Committee on National Health Promotion and Disease Prevention Objectives for 2020 (HHS, 2009).

BOX 2-1
On Scorecards

The term *scorecards* is sometimes used to refer to health-indicator sets that provide a snapshot of an area's health (for example, How is X County compared with a national standard, compared with Y County in a given state, or compared with last year?). However, the term's specific meaning in the business, education, and clinical care settings—as a tool for internal performance evaluation (for example, balanced scorecards)—is different from the meaning and purpose of many health-indicator sets. The committee struggled with achieving clarity about the seemingly overlapping meanings of the terms used in measurement and recognized that the purposes of performance measurement, public reporting, and mobilization are not necessarily independent or neatly separate from one another. The lack of semantic exactness regarding health indicators has led to a conflation of two primary meanings: "measures of health" and "measures of performance on health." Many public health or population health data sets (as opposed to data sets used in the clinical care context) called scorecards or report cards are not, in fact, intended for or capable of measuring the performance of public health agencies in a county or state, of other organizations, or of communities in general. The committee discusses this difficulty with use of the term *scorecard* further in Chapter 4, "Measurement and Accountability."

---

quarterly measure of gross domestic product. In this chapter and throughout much of the report, the committee will use the term *indicators* to denote components of data sets that convey information (comparative or ranked) about the health status of the country, states, and counties. *Indicators* will also refer to a variety of existing and potential metrics used to inform, mobilize, and advocate and in the context of a later discussion of measurement in accountability (in Chapter 4).[3] The term *scorecards* is used to refer to some of these efforts and their indicator sets (see Box 2-1 and Chapter 4 for a discussion of this term).

---

[3] On the difference between performance measures and outcome measures: The two types of measures may overlap in terminology and operationally. In ideal circumstances, it would be easy to draw a straight line between cause and effect in population health, elucidating a clear causal relationship between system inputs, such as programs or policies, and system outputs, such as health outcomes. Sufficient resources and other capabilities would be deployed in interventions supported by evidence, best practices, or strong theoretical arguments and would move public health agencies and their partners in the direction of achieving desired outcomes. However, health is the result of complex and dynamic interactions, data on which are often lacking. Because the evidence needed to elucidate the pathway from specific inputs to a given output is often incomplete, decisions as to which data to collect are challenging, and it is often difficult to collect the needed data. This is a topic in which research and analysis, including predictive and systems modeling, can help to elucidate the causal pathways, fill gaps in knowledge, and inform a variety of decision-making and policy-making.

THE NEED FOR A DETERMINANTS-OF-HEALTH PERSPECTIVE

Strengthening the usefulness of the population health information system requires integrating the concept of social and environmental determinants of health (discussed in detail in Chapter 1) and adopting a population-based approach to improving health in all data-collection efforts and in the highest level of strategic planning for the statistics and information enterprise. Figures 2-1a and 2-1b illustrate the population health and clinical care approaches to the sample outcomes of infant mortality and cardiovascular disease (CVD). The figures depict how interventions and the stakeholders involved in two or more health outcomes may overlap and are intended to show a broader view of how population health is created (including but going well beyond clinical care). In the figures, clinical care delivery system interventions are depicted on the left (in blue) and interventions or actions rooted in the ecologic–multiple-determinants perspective on the right (in green). As examples of the capacity of ecologic, population-based approaches to influence multiple health outcomes, some domains or stakeholders with potential multiple (and overlapping) effects are highlighted (in orange).

Successful strategies for improving both infant and cardiovascular health require complementary interventions in multiple sectors to promote the desired change through the feedback loops that connect them. Of note are the synergies associated with combating the vastly different problems of infant mortality and CVD when the interventions are generated through a population health model. In moving from the left side of a figure toward the right side, one is reminded of the shift in the public health community's perspective of the "actual causes of death," traced in the work of McGinnis and Foege (1993) and later Mokdad and colleagues (2004), from a largely biomedical-model perspective (for example, with respect to heart disease, cancer, and stroke) to one that recognizes upstream causes, including unhealthy behaviors (for example, tobacco use, inadequate physical activity, poor nutrition, and alcohol abuse) and the environmental conditions that may precipitate them. Given the strong and compelling evidence of broad social and economic influences on health, contemporary researchers describe an even more upstream set of causes of death and poor health. It is highlighted in the work of the Robert Wood Johnson Commission to Build a Healthier America (2009) and the commission's high-profile messages that place matters and that the influence of ZIP codes (and the socioeconomic environments they represent) outweighs that of genetic codes. The actual causes of death as understood today could be described as place of residence, socioeconomic status, income inequality, discrimination, and other policy and environmental factors (see, for example, Braveman and Egerter, 2008; Egerter et al., 2009).

Although the importance of the upstream factors is widely recognized

39

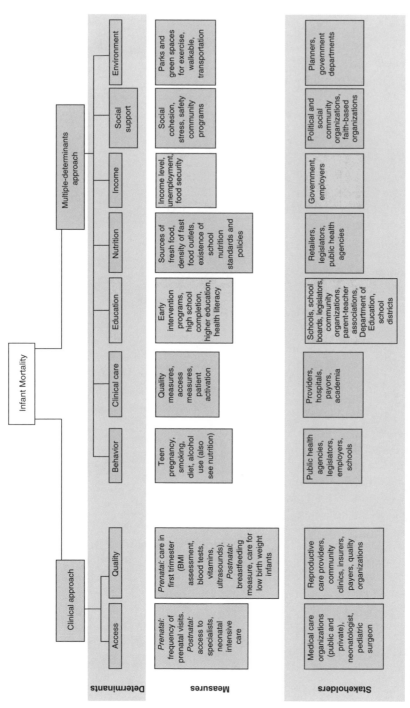

FIGURE 2-1a Contrasting the multiple-determinants and clinical approaches to addressing infant mortality.

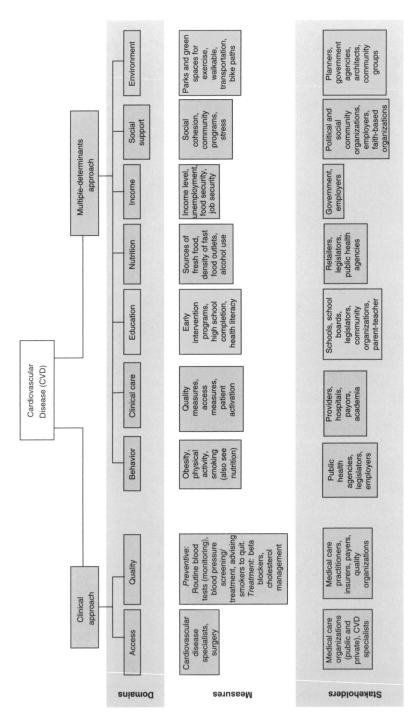

FIGURE 2-1b Contrasting the multiple-determinants and clinical approaches to addressing cardiovascular disease.

and is a subject of growing scientific research, local decision-makers who wish to assess these factors often find it difficult to do so because of lack of data. At the national and state levels, where more data are available on some determinants of health, such as income and poverty, the problem may be not a lack of data but the existence of "multiple data bases, multiple estimates, and uncertainty about which survey produces the best numbers" (O'Grady, 2006). The lack of accurate local data on social, environmental, and behavioral determinants of health not only impedes policy action but also obscures basic awareness of the issue and leaves the public uninformed about important trends. A common presumption is that health is defined by clinical care. How health really is improved and disease prevented or controlled remains largely invisible to most Americans, owing in large part to a failure to convey this information to the public. Although many organizations, individuals, and groups in communities all around the country are engaged in activities intended to target various aspects of the determinants of health—including employment, education, housing, access to healthy food, early childhood interventions, safe communities, livable (walkable and accessible) communities, and fair labor standards—the linkages among these activities and their influence on the broader health and well-being of communities are often not made. Inadequacies in public awareness of what creates good health and, in turn, the benefits of good health itself (such as greater potential for economic productivity and prosperity) can be addressed partially by the availability of reliable information about local health outcomes and their determinants and by an effective strategy to communicate the information to the public and decision-makers.

Multiple factors influence a population's health heavily, but the United States, unlike its neighbor Canada, lacks a systematic national strategy to identify and address the set of social and environmental determinants of health that are most responsible for health outcomes. Several European countries have for many decades collected health data according to detailed socioeconomic categories—for example, from income rankings to occupational hierarchies (Braveman et al., 2010). Recent Canadian and British examples include the *Canadian Senate Report on the Determinants of Health* (Mikkonen and Raphael, 2010) and the report *Fair Society, Healthy Lives: A Strategic Review of Health Inequalities in England Post-2010* (The Marmot Review, 2010). The Affordable Care Act of 2010 (ACA) includes components that pertain to population health and refers to the "social and primary determinants of health" (Public Law 111-148), but the national dialogue and federal activities that both preceded and have followed the act's passage have not done enough to advance public understanding of the non-medical-care-related contributors to the health of Americans, such as housing, built and natural environments, income, education, occupation, culture, inequity, and discrimination. However, there are recent examples of the federal government's recognition of the importance of integrating a determinants-of-health perspective into the process of rethinking and exploring innovative changes in data collection. For example, "in 2009, the Centers for Disease Control and Prevention (CDC), through the Behavioral Risk Factor Surveillance System (BRFSS), introduced a 'social context' module, which is being used by 12 states, the District of Columbia, and 20 communities and consists of eight questions intended to assess civic engagement and food, housing, and job security" (Friedman and Parrish, 2009b).

Despite a long history of efforts to prepare a national report on social (and cultural) indicators to measure progress and inform policy, the United States lacks such an accounting (GAO, 2004). In the 1960s, there were several attempts to prepare a national document on social indicators, beginning with the *Social Indicators* report prepared by the American Academy of Arts and Sciences (at the request of a federal agency) (GAO, 2004) and the 1969 publication from the Department of Health, Education, and Welfare (DHEW)[4] titled *Toward a Social Report* (Department of Health, Education, and Welfare, 1969). According to a Government Accountability Office (GAO) report (2004), the DHEW document concluded that "indicators on social and cultural conditions were lacking, and recommended that the executive branch prepare a comprehensive social report for the nation with emphasis on indicators to measure social change that could be used in setting policy and goals." In the 1970s and early 1980s, both federal and academic or nonprofit efforts in this subject continued, but no major centralized national or federal effort was established and sustained. (The new National Prevention, Health Promotion, and Public Health Council created by the ACA offers an opportunity for a "health in all" approach to population health improvement that potentially could involve interdepartmental attention to the underlying causes of poor health in the United States.[5])

A report by the Department of Health and Human Services (HHS) and NCHS, *Health, United States, 1998,* had a special focus on socioeconomic status and health (NCHS, 1998). Although a small subset of socioeconomic factors have been addressed in its annual updates, HHS has not made an examination of an array of health-outcomes data by socioeconomic variables a major theme since 1998. Several other federal documents focus on subjects related to determinants of health, including the series of annual Agency for Healthcare Research and Quality (AHRQ) *National Healthcare Disparities Reports* and the National Health Interview Survey Series 10 reports (AHRQ, 2007; CDC, 2010). However, the former

---

[4] Predecessor of today's HHS.

[5] The health-in-all-policies approach refers to crosscutting analyses that examine ramifications of all types of policy decisions for health outcomes by using such tools as health impact assessments. This approach is used extensively in Europe, and to some extent in the United States.

focus on medical care, and the latter do not consider race and economic factors in combination (Braveman et al., 2010). Aside from those efforts, the United States does not have a federally led national-level annual report on the socioeconomic and environmental determinants of health.[6] There have been several academic and nonprofit efforts to fill the gap in recent years. In 1999, sociologists Marc Miringoff and Marque-Luisa Miringoff published *The Social Health of the Nation: How America Is Really Doing*, which put forward an Index of Social Health, an effort that has not been sustained (Miringoff and Miringoff, 1999). More recently, the Social Science Research Council created the American Human Development Project, which publishes the annual report *Measure of America* (Burd-Sharpe et al., 2010), and the Virginia Commonwealth University established its *Center on Human Needs,* which gathers and communicates data on societal distress[7] (Virginia Commonwealth University, 2009).

There is growing recognition of the importance of incorporating the determinants of health in the broadest strategies for health-data collection and for implementing effective policies to improve public health. What remains absent is a concerted and systematic effort to capture relevant data on the determinants and to make them easily accessible to policy-makers in ways that are useful for making decisions, especially at the state and local levels. The committee believes that this activity is most appropriately located within the federal government in an effort to gather and report data on health determinants, including disparities, which could serve as a compelling tool for informing Americans and mobilizing action.

RESPONSIVENESS TO THE NEEDS OF END USERS

Committee members heard about the data needs of communities and local decision-makers in its information-gathering sessions and at other meetings (IOM, 2010b), such as a launch meeting hosted by the Institute of Medicine (IOM) for HHS's Community Health Data Initiative (CHDI), which has served as a platform for publicizing the HHS Data Warehouse operated by NCHS. Multiple participants asked about the availability of local (for example, county, ZIP code, and census-tract) data and learned that most of the federal population health data available currently lack that level of specificity.

From the perspective of end users, such as local decision-makers in general and public health officials in particular, efforts must be made to improve the characteristics of available data, particularly completeness,

---

[6] The Davos Conference report on competitiveness shows that the United States lags in determinants of health, signaling potentially worsening health outcomes in the future (Schwab et al., 2010).

[7] Societal distress is measured in five domains: food, housing, health, education, and income.

usefulness, geographic relevance, and timeliness. The information needed by end users resides in different administrative structures, and the data are often not readily accessible. Federal activity, state and local contributions, and independent supplements to data collection could be enhanced by a more integrated approach overseen by a central body that more fully ascertains and addresses state and local needs (such as sample design, populations included, and health issues measured).

Since the middle 1990s, federal health-statistics programs, such as the CDC National Health Interview Survey (NHIS) and the AHRQ Medical Expenditure Panel Survey, have made great strides in increasing the timeliness of reporting of data collected and, through partnerships with nonprofit organizations, have improved their ability to provide state and local data (Academy Health, 2004). Although there has been a consistent trend toward timeliness and local usefulness of federal data, gaps remain because of resource limitations and other factors that are detailed below.

Data are partly or largely lacking on some indicators that are needed to inform decisions and action, including environmental monitoring data (Luck et al., 2006); chronic-disease prevalence and prevention or control (Goff et al., 2007a; Luck et al., 2006), with asthma as one example (Mendez-Luck et al., 2007) and diabetes another (Goff et al., 2007b); data on health behaviors, such as tobacco use; and data on aspects of the built environment, such as housing quality—for example, the Census Bureau's American Housing Survey collects data every 6 years on housing quality in metropolitan areas, but few data are available on small areas or neighborhoods in some jurisdictions (Krieger and Higgins, 2002).

The existing sets of indicators generally were not designed to convey information that can identify loci for intervention to improve health. They are therefore unable to provide actionable insights on health that a local official can put to use. There are also critical gaps in information where the evidence base suggests a relationship between a given determinant and an intermediate or distal outcome, but the methods of capturing or representing that determinant validly and reliably are not yet developed. In such a case, use of multiple, disconnected health indicators may not provide the appropriate guidance for population-based strategies for which understanding of causal pathways between conditions and exposures and intermediate and distal health outcomes is critical.

Communities and decision-makers need data that provide useful information for judging the health of communities. It is crucial that the population health statistics and information system adopt as its core mission serving decision-makers, not simply compiling or analyzing statistics or serving national-level planning needs. The system, and especially its federal-government core, must determine what kinds of information are needed at the community level (through broad consultation); ensure that such data are collected (both primary collection as items on population surveys and secondary aggregation from all relevant public and private sources into databases and warehouses), updated, vetted for quality, and made accessible to users in terms of both ease of access and localization to the community level; and elicit feedback on completeness, usefulness, timeliness, and geographic relevance of data in a feedback loop to the first step. One important need is for a generic measure of health status (for example, health-adjusted life expectancy or the equivalent) because disease-specific statistics are not sufficient. The population health statistics and information system is producing a surplus of data and indicators that are not all conducive to the assessment of health. Through its CHDI and its NCHS-managed HHS Health Indicators Warehouse, HHS has made great strides in making its data more useful to the public by beginning to develop interactive interfaces and front ends that serve the needs of users. This ambitious effort to make an array of federal health data widely available (HHS, 2010a) and integrate them with additional federal data sources on factors that influence health, such as the US Department of Agriculture Food Environment Atlas, is intended to inform the development of independent and potentially health-supporting applications by multiple private-sector and public-sector (local government) programmers and others (HHS, 2010b). However, more is needed—for example, to develop mechanisms for collecting systematic decision-maker and public input on the data and on current and projected user needs.

In general, the availability of statistical data decreases as one moves from the national level to the state level and then to the local level (see Figure 2-2 and description below for more detail). Some federal data provide only national-level information, and there are challenges to developing small-area estimates. Several changes could help, including additional methodologic research; the use of technologic innovations to facilitate rapid, inexpensive, and effective local data collection; and changes in national data-collection efforts to replace obsolete or less useful components with components of local relevance. Attention to the needs of federal statistical efforts in this endeavor is exemplified by the 2009 NCHS Board of Scientific Counselors programmatic review of the National Health and Nutrition Examination Survey (NHANES), which urged NCHS to explore "potential ways to improve the cost efficiency and screening efficiency for area probability sample recruitment by utilizing commercial data bases for household enumeration" and called for exploring the possibilities for integrating the design of NHIS and NHANES—a recommendation made by others (NCHS, 2009).

The US vital statistics system provides an example of several persisting challenges. It is a decentralized system: localities collect data that are then compiled by states and submitted to NCHS. However, in recent years, delays in the availability of data have been caused by the combination of aging collection systems (including inadequate automation) and a change

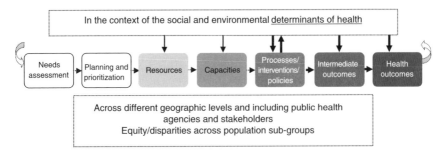

FIGURE 2-2 From inputs to outputs logic model.
NOTE: The thickness of some arrows denotes the present report's focus on those interactions.

in standards (Rothwell et al., 2004). For example, state registrars reporting vital statistics to NCHS may have to wait up to 3 years to get analyzed and usable data back; this constitutes a persistent lag in federal-agency reporting (caused in large part by systemic challenges arising from the multiple state and county collection mechanisms involved). In the interim, state and local public health agencies may be constrained by federal statutes in their ability to use preliminary data (Starr and Starr, 1995; personal communication, S. Teutsch, October 2010). Some federal data-collection entities, such as the Census Bureau, have made strides in improving access to current data, and private sources (such as Google) often are able to make data available quickly.

To address the challenges of incompleteness and less than optimal use-fulness (including geographic relevance and timeliness), end users would benefit from the establishment of more formalized processes that allow local and state high-priority needs to be identified and aligned with data capture at the national level. There is often a mismatch between federal health-statistical objectives and the needs of local jurisdictions, and little progress has been made to date in reconciling the different perspectives and ensuring that local and state public health officials can obtain sufficient informa-tion to guide priority-setting and other decisions. Each of the three major federally supported population health statistics efforts—BRFSS, NHIS, and NHANES—has its strengths and weaknesses (see discussion in Appendix B), but they do not, collectively, fully meet the information needs of local decision-makers and communities (for example, BRFSS generally does not allow sub-state-level estimates, and NHANES does not contain state-specific data). In addition, the federal and state efforts are not harmonized to maxi-mize the use of resources and realize other efficiencies. In summary, the com-mittee identifies two facts that present a serious challenge to coordination and integration across geographic levels:

1. "Top-down" federal data-collection efforts often rely on samples designed to produce national or regional estimates and therefore are not designed to collect geographically based samples large enough to support reliable estimates and comparisons at the community level.
2. "Bottom-up" state and local data-collection efforts often are not standardized and coordinated with each other and with federal efforts so as to support concatenation ("rollup") and valid comparisons among communities.

The solution involves standardization and coordination. Two examples of bottom-up coordination and standardization that work are the AHRQ Healthcare Cost and Utilization Project, which standardizes and combines all-payer hospital-discharge data collected by 43 states and thereby allows local estimates and comparisons (Healthcare Cost and Utilization Project, 2010), and state cancer registries, which have improved standardization through accreditation certification (National Program of Cancer Registries, 2010).

Research, Modeling, and Other Capabilities Needed to "Translate" Data into Indicators That Can Inform Decision-Makers

The 2009 National Research Council report on principles and practices for federal statistical agencies outlines a broader potential role for such an agency as NCHS, including a more extensive role in research (NRC, 2009). A revitalized NCHS could provide leadership for the entire population health statistics and information enterprise (the diverse array of public and private producers, analyzers, and conveyors of population health data) by contributing to coordination and collaboration among government (and private-sector) entities to conduct or support extensive analyses and research, including indicator development and predictive and systems-based modeling to improve understanding of the relationships between the determinants of health and specific health outcomes, to inform cost-effectiveness advice for decision-makers, and to meet other needs.

Timely and authoritative review of the evidence base for the relationships between prominent indicators and population health outcomes is needed to ensure that indicators reflect contemporary understanding of determinants of health. For example, logic models, such as those in the *Guide to Community Preventive Services,* are needed to link indicators to actions or interventions and the evidence that supports them. Government and other data-collection efforts, such as population-based surveys, can be improved through regular review, methodologic improvements, and other changes. Although NCHS data-collection efforts are periodically reviewed, the agency lacks the resources needed to implement necessary changes and to conduct more frequent and extensive reviews (for example, to seek broader input from local users and from people who have relevant methodologic expertise). In 2008 and 2009, the NCHS Board of Scientific Counselors conducted program reviews of NHIS and NHANES (NCHS, 2008, 2009). Both reviews identified severe resource and staff limitations, difficulties in meeting state and local health-information needs, and methodologic challenges and opportunities requiring more in-depth research.

The committee recognizes the extraordinary complexity of causal pathways in population health and the need to advance the science, through observational studies and such tools as modeling (discussed below and in Chapter 3), to understand the effects of determinants on each other (Lahelma et al., 2004), to elucidate the relationships between various inputs, intermediate outcomes, and distal (population health) outcomes, and to improve understanding of the potential effects of various options that may be considered by policy-makers.

Commonly used criteria to evaluate indicators include methodologic soundness (validity, reliability, and whether collected over a long period), feasibility (available or collectable), meaningfulness (Is the measure linked to an evidence-based intervention, and is it relevant and actionable?), and importance (Is it an important outcome, and is the outcome linked to evidence-based interventions?). As one example, studies of the food environment[8] and individual access to healthy foods include a variety of indicators to measure community and individual access, but there is little agreement about which indicators are most useful on the basis of the criteria above. Indicators used include distance from one's home to the nearest retailer of healthy and affordable foods, walkable distance to a grocery store (0.5 miles is used in urban areas), level of choice (for example, access to three chain supermarkets), ratio of fast-food outlets to supermarkets in a given area, and number of supermarkets (or fast-food restaurants or convenience stores) per resident. An example of the complexity that researchers encounter is found in attempts to use the distance from one's residence to a store as a measure of access. However, assuming that people travel from home to the grocery store would lead to an underestimation of access in that people often incorporate food shopping in other trips, such as travel to work and school (Ver Ploeg et al., 2009).

The committee believes that the field could be advanced through the development of a research agenda on developing useful, high-quality indicators. For many kinds of measurement, including measurements in the

---

[8] The term *food deserts* has been brought into public consciousness by recent federal government efforts to address the increasing problem of overweight and obesity, and it is used to refer to geographic areas severely underserved by food retailers that sell fresh food, such as fruits and vegetables (see, for example,Ver Ploeg et al., 2009).

realm of the determinants of health (such as quality of housing, social co-hesion, and access to healthy foods), there is much ambiguity about what indicators should be used and how they should be developed or selected for specific purposes. Some measures or indicators are more precise than oth-ers or have better validation, documentation, and evidence of performance characteristics. In educational attainment, for example, multiple indicators are available, but there is little evidence to help in differentiating among them and selecting the best ones. Indicators include highest level of school-ing completed in adults 25 years old and older, percentage of high school graduates, proportion of 9th graders who complete high school, proportion of 25-year-olds with a high school diploma or an equivalent, and average grade attained. Measures of other critical educational characteristics, such as health literacy, are even less well developed. The creation of a reposi-tory or clearinghouse to hold and disseminate the best knowledge in health measurement could help to address the uncertainty about which measures are best for the various determinants of health.

NEED FOR IMPROVED COORDINATION AT THE NATIONAL LEVEL (INCLUDING FEDERAL AGENCIES)

NCHS and several other HHS agencies produce much of the population health data used by academic researchers, public-sector and nonprofit col-laborations, and many others, including a variety of local jurisdictions, to develop or adapt indicator sets that they track and regularly report on to the public. Many data sets and information streams feed into the health system, but the committee asserts that the population health statistics and infor-mation enterprise has limitations in the content (for example, useful data and measures available for monitoring progress), processes, integration, and coordination necessary to maximize its usefulness to the promotion of public health and to inform the contributions of multiple stakeholders in the system. Data are required by decision-makers and other users so that they can understand the health of particular populations (by geographic level or sociodemographic community), make informed decisions on interventions to improve health outcomes, and assess whether the actions taken are hav-ing the desired effects.

Although HHS statistical tools, such as surveys, and relevant methods are reviewed and updated, existing processes are not sufficiently extensive, frequent, or forward-looking, in large part because of severe resource and staff constraints (for one example of resource constraints pertaining to NCHS, see NCHS, 2008, 2009). On a practical level, forms, rules, and unwieldy or non-user-friendly Web interfaces often make it difficult to ac-cess what government data are available. Although statutory and ethical requirements are essential, it is possible to streamline and rationalize the data that are available, and efforts have been undertaken to address some of these challenges; the HHS Gateway to Data and Statistics provides an example (HHS, 2010d). The need for increased coordination is evident in the current state of health data; the proliferation of data sets in the absence of common, standardized health-outcome indicators (indicators of distal health outcomes, such as disease rates, and intermediate outcomes, such as hypertension) and indicators of community health (not aggregate measures of individual health outcomes, such as cause-specific mortality and morbidity, but true measures of a community's intrinsic healthfulness and well-being); the multiple agencies and groups collecting data often in isolation of one another; the lack of processes for aligning local and state information needs with data collection by federal agencies; and the lack of processes for periodically reviewing and replacing obsolete data elements and meeting changing needs and circumstances.

Better coordination is needed to address a cluster of related issues, including operational inefficiencies; the lack of agreed-on standard indicators or indicator sets that can be used to inform population health efforts at all levels (and thus transcend the proliferation of indicator sets); the lack of optimal coordination and linkage among sectors (for example, data sources in the public and private sectors); inadequate strategic planning for the future (for example, future population health information needs); and the lack of research on the characteristics and purposes of measures (how they link to processes or outcomes) and of a current, readily available clearinghouse for indicators. (The challenges regarding standardization and connectivity resemble those faced by the vast national investment in electronic health records.)

The absence of a common framework or core set of indicators for a given domain makes it difficult for decision-makers and health-system collaborators at each level (local, state, and national) to have a comprehensive, coherent, consistent, and meaningful top-to-bottom view of the status of and change in health over time (Bilheimer, 2010).

In its discussion about existing indicators and the need for indicators, the committee used a schematic, or logic model, of the steps to population health improvement, from inputs to outputs (for example, distal health outcomes). Numerous logic models are available to depict population health efforts and public health practice (see, for example, BARHII and PHLP, 2010; County Health Ranking, 2010; Kindig et al., 2008; Parrish, 2010; Secretary's Advisory Committee on National Health Promotion and Disease Prevention Objectives for 2020, 2010). The committee adapted a simple structure–process–outcome logic model (Donabedian, 1988) to illustrate both the sequence of steps between inputs and outputs in population health and the multiple categories for measurement (see Figure 2-2).[9]

Although developed with awareness of the limitations of a simple, largely linear model, the committee's figure is provided to help in thinking about the types of data and indicators available and needed at each step in the process. The steps in the figure extend from resources and capabilities to intermediate outcomes and indicators and distal outcomes. The increasingly dark shading of the boxes shows where more indicators are available in public health. Generally, more measures are available as one moves toward the right side of the figure (intermediate and health outcomes), and far fewer measures are available for resources, capacities, and processes (and from the national level to the local). A different way to illustrate this is to focus on the level of user (for example, national, state, and local). In Table 2-1— which gives sample measures of obesity, smoking, and infant mortality—the availability of useful data and information decreases as one moves from the national to the local level and from left to right (from measures of interventions, processes, and policies to health outcomes). The determinants-of-health box in Figure 2-2 is intended to refer largely to determinants that can be modified by the actions of various agencies and organization in the health system. Such determinants as genetic factors are less amenable to the influence of system actors. Arrows between the determinants of health and many of the boxes represent the feedback loops between determinants and system inputs or outputs. For example, broader societal values and priorities influence the availability of resources for population health activities. Population health interventions, such as policy changes, are often designed to influence particular determinants of health. After evaluation and research to assess the effectiveness of an intervention on a given determinant, the intervention may be modified or replaced.

Some indicators are available to show changes in some of the antecedents of health, but they are largely measures of behavioral risk (such as smoking rates). (However, even data of this kind are incomplete, because national surveys do not provide information on "awareness, detection, treatment, and control of physical inactivity, unhealthy diet, cigarette

---

[9] The classic model for assessing quality of care put forth by Donabedian includes structure, process, and outcomes. Structure is defined as "the attributes of the settings in which care occurs," including resources (money), human resources (personnel), and organization structure. Process refers to what is actually implemented, and outcomes are the effects of what was implemented on the health status of patients and populations. According to Donabedian's model, processes are constrained by the structures in which they operate, and good processes lead to good outcomes. Donabedian notes that this relationship must be established before any component of the model (structure, process, outcomes) can be used to assess quality and that "there must be preexisting knowledge of the linkage between structure and process, and between process and outcome, before quality assessment can be undertaken" (Donabedian, 1988, p. 1745).

TABLE 2-1 Measures Related to Obesity, Smoking, and Infant Mortality

Geographic Level	Measures of Interventions, Processes, and Policies	Measures of Intermediate Outcomes or Determinants	Measures of (Distal) Health Outcomes
National • Public health agencies and stakeholders	• Food labeling • Federal cigarette-tax increase	• Obesity rates • Smoking rates; number of cigarettes smoked per day	• Diabetes rates • Years of life lost because of smoking • Lung-cancer deaths • Cardiovascular disease (CVD) rates
		• Prenatal insurance coverage	• Infant mortality and premature birth
State • Public health agencies and stakeholders	• Trans-fat ban • State cigarette-tax increase	• Obesity rates • Number of cigarettes smoked per day	• Diabetes rates • CVD rates
		• Frequency of prenatal visits	• Infant mortality and premature birth
Local • Public health agencies and stakeholders	• Removing sodas from vending machines • Smoking-cessation programs offered to employees • Free or low-cost prenatal care in community clinics	• Walkability (miles of sidewalk vs. miles of roads) • Use of antismoking campaigns • Maternal smoking	• Diabetes rates • Deaths from smoking-related illnesses • Infant mortality and premature births

NOTE: The boundaries between categories are not always clear. For example, obesity rates may function as a measure of intermediate outcomes (a risk factor) or as a health outcome in its own right. Some measures of intermediate outcomes may also function as measures of community health, such as measures of walkability and recreational space.

smoking, and obesity" (Goff et al., 2007a). Few data are available on an array of determinants of health (exceptions include education and income data, for which robust national and state statistics are available), and even fewer are available at the most local level (for example, census-tract data on educational attainment, income, and clean air) that could inform decision-makers and communities and that may be influenced by population-level interventions (for example, to support high school completion, to ensure a living wage, and to reduce carbon emissions). Measures of performance (that capture the effectiveness of efforts of the health system broadly and of public health agencies specifically) are also less available; this is discussed in more detail in Chapter 4.

A Wealth of Indicators

Recent years have seen rapid development of a number of health-indicator sets that are based on data made available by federal agencies and other organizations. One of the higher-profile sets is found in the series of Healthy People initiatives from HHS. Healthy People 2010 (HP 2010) included a set of leading health indicators (it is pertinent to the above discussion that none of these was an indicator of social determinants of health) (HHS, 2010c).[10] Despite the use of the availability of measures as one criterion for selecting the leading health indicators, the measures used to assess that progress are often inadequate representations. For example, the measures for environmental quality are exposure to secondhand smoke and air pollution as assessed on the basis of ozone concentration. The HP 2020 process began in 2009 (HHS, 2009); in fall 2010, a new IOM committee was formed to identify lead objectives and health indicators for HP 2020 (IOM, 2010a).

The indicator sets and calls to action are valuable tools, and careful thinking and effort have gone into the creation of parsimonious sets of indicators that draw from data currently collected through federal and state initiatives. They include the Community Health Status Indicators and the County Health Rankings (Mobilizing Action Toward Community Health) at the local level and America's Health Rankings and the State of the USA (SUSA) measures at the state level (and for SUSA, the national and potentially the county level) (Community Health Status Indicators, 2009; SUSA, 2010; University of Wisconsin Population Health Institute, 2010).

The SUSA activity is noteworthy because its 20-indicator set was developed by an IOM committee after a long process of collaboration between the GAO and the National Academies, a process culminating in the ACA's provisions for a system of key national indicators to be managed by the

---

[10] HP 2010 leading health indicators included physical activity, overweight and obesity, tobacco use, substance abuse, responsible sexual behavior, mental health, injury and violence, environmental quality, immunization, and access to health care (HHS, 2010c).

National Academies (IOM, 2008). The implementation of the provision is still in the very early stage; final appointments and appropriations have not yet been made. However, if a set of key health indicators for the nation is adopted, either drawing on the existing IOM-developed health set of the SUSA key indicators or using a different standardized set, such an action could potentially facilitate a solution to the problem of too many disconnected sets. However, other kinds of standardization are also needed (for example, with respect to education and income) because other measures will be needed to capture the effects of all sectors on health and to reflect changes over time. Trust for America's Health also develops regular ranking reports on state health issues, including expenditures and emergency preparedness (Trust for America's Health, 2010). In the realm of medical care, the Commonwealth Fund issues annual national scorecards "on U.S. health system performance" (Commonwealth Fund, 2009). Various other sets of health-status indicators are available, and a wide array of organizations—including clinical care quality entities, local governments and local public health agencies, and private-sector groups—issue regular or sporadic reports on health and clinical care.[11] Examples include the Take Care New York program, which reports on 10 select indicators (Summers et al., 2009), and Seattle–King County's Communities Count (Seattle and King County Public Health Department, 2010).

Other current indicator efforts focus more generally on aspects of well-being (of which health is often a dimension) and involve nonprofit, academic, and government-based actors. A nonprofit example is the Urban Institute's National Neighborhood Indicators Partnership (GAO, 2004; Luck et al., 2006). The Federal Interagency Forum on Child and Family Statistics produces an annual report on the well-being of American children—for example, *America's Children in Brief: Key National Indicators of Well-Being, 2010* (Federal Interagency Forum on Child and Family Statistics, 2010).[12]

Appendix B provides more detailed descriptions of the small array of health-indicator sets listed above. The committee did not attempt to prepare a comprehensive and systematic catalog or evaluation of all activities (national, state, and local) that put forth health indicators or indicators of well-being. However, the committee refers to two overviews of indicator efforts in the health field (Public Health Institute, 2010; Wold, 2008) and a

---

[11] See, for example, the Gallup–Healthways Well-Being Index, an interesting effort to gather self-reported data on six dimensions of life that aggregates and reports by month self-reported data that are collected daily on life situation, emotional health, physical health, healthy behavior, work environment, and basic access (to life's necessities) (Gallup–Healthways, 2008).

[12] In its review of the literature, the committee also became aware of the Environmental Defense Scorecard pollution-information site that provides data by ZIP code and a variety of indicator sets in other fields, such as education (see, for example, the No Child Left Behind measurement efforts).

more general summary of key indicators (on multiple topics beyond health, including the economy, society, and the environment) in the GAO report *Informing Our Nation: Improving How to Understand and Assess the USA's Position and Progress* (GAO, 2004).

Those many activities clearly are responsive to the need to capture and report information that can prompt understanding and action at local, state, and national levels and can serve as benchmarks or sentinel indicators to spur further investigation and knowledge development. Growth in the number of indicator sets (by one estimate, there are more than 100 indicator projects at the national, state, and local levels [Rudolph, 2009]) and of individual indicators within a set on similar subjects may cause confusion, is inefficient, and impairs valid comparisons. The proliferation and heterogeneity of indicator sets can overwhelm busy decision-makers; a consistent set is needed to provide information that can be used to guide population health actions in the health system. Measurement strategies that are consistent among communities are also central to advancing the health of the public. Currently, different communities use different information sources, and this limits the ability to compare communities, establish benchmarks, and understand reasons for differences.

Boufford and Lee (2001) outlined the HHS challenge of fragmentation and lack of coordination among 212 separate departmental data systems in existence at the beginning of the decade and emphasized that most of the data collection by the department focused on a small proportion of the determinants of health, specifically, on infectious agents and medical treatments. The 2002 document *Shaping a Health Statistics Vision for the 21st Century,* a major federal-government document on the "health-statistics enterprise," also described multiple panels and activities and a lack of coordination within the department, pointing out that "multiple initiatives and forums themselves add to the perception of fragmentation and disorganization in the overall health statistics enterprise" (HHS et al., 2002). Other researchers have shown that there are numerous incentives for federal funders to support the creation of program-specific public health information systems and that this has led to the proliferation of multiple stand-alone information systems—for example, immunization registries and large-city National Electronic Disease Surveillance Systems separate from those developed by states (Friedman et al., 2005; Lumpkin and Richards, 2002; Safran et al., 2007). Similar reasons (such as the urgency of filling infrastructure gaps) explain the lack of coordination between county and state information systems and the fact that federal funders are not always able to provide incentives for greater coordination (Lumpkin and Richards, 2002).

Data-collection processes in federal agencies and at state and local levels have generally evolved in isolation from one another (Brownson et al., 2010); information on measurement of the upstream determinants of health remains modest (Brownson et al., 2010); and even when there is a good understanding of measures of a particular risk factor or outcome, they are often not available at the requisite level of timeliness (Bilheimer, 2010), detail, or specificity: for example, measures of cardiovascular mortality and, in some cases, the prevalence of CVD and obesity are available locally, but the prevalence of hypertension and data on lipid concentrations are usually unavailable, as are measures of physical activity or nutritional status and habits (Goff et al., 2007a).

Linking to Other Sources of Data

In its 2010 concept paper, the National Committee on Vital and Health Statistics (NCVHS), a federal advisory committee to the secretary of HHS staffed by NCHS, observed that "new investments in electronic health records (EHRs) and health information exchanges are important contributors, especially for clinical care, but the benefits from these investments will be limited unless the synergies with other types of health information are recognized and used" (NCVHS, 2010). The report also asked for "inclusion not just of traditional health-related data, but also of data on the full array of determinants of health, including community attributes and cultural context" (NCVHS, 2010).

The 2002 HHS vision of the future of health statistics similarly noted that the "current health statistics enterprise lacks the ability to develop and articulate effective positions and to engage with the producers of non-health sources of data that is important to understanding health, and also lacks the ability to effectively pursue opportunities to use data that flow from these other producers" (HHS et al., 2002). In their review of implementation of the 2002 vision, Friedman and Parrish (2009a) found that expert key informants (including NCHS staff and former and current NCVHS members) believed that the health-information technology effort in medical care had had little or no effect on the population health statistics enterprise despite the 2002 recommendation urging exploration of ways to integrate personal clinical care data with other information streams. The limited interaction with the private sector may be due to the staff and resource limitations highlighted in NCHS program reviews and by others (see, for example, Population Association of America, 2010). However, EHRs and other data sources can both complement and be enriched by linkages to population health data.

In addition to the rich stores of data available in HHS and other government agencies—and efforts are under way to make them more accessible to the public, under the Open Government Directive (Executive Office of the President, 2009)—other data needed for population health assessment reside in the private sector, and in many cases there is no established mechanism for sharing such data with the public sector, with communities, and with other stakeholders to yield novel and potentially useful insights. Other examples of domains of community-health measures and data sources include crime and safety (data could include injury surveys available from public health agencies and other data from law-enforcement agencies and private-sector neighborhood crime-tracking programs and could be used to assess the effect of state and local gun-control laws and community policing activities); healthy housing (a subdomain of the built environment, on which data could include results of lead screening by public health agencies and data from the Department of Housing and Urban Development and other agency housing surveys, information from developers and real-estate databases, and free online sources, all of which could be linked to census-tract pre-1970 housing and school test scores); and transportation (public health agency data on bicycle use, pedestrians, and injuries; data from the Department of Transportation; and private-sector data on commercial bus, rail, and other transit—all of which could be used to assess the effect of helmet-use laws).

The examples above show how data potentially available from the private sector could be used to augment information available from public agencies and, in some cases, be the exclusive basis of key information about factors that influence health in a community. Indeed, other sectors have often developed and validated useful indicators. For example, banking institutions and financial-service companies may use the local ratio of full-service banks to check-cashing facilities as a proxy measure of economic development or at least of financial access in neighborhoods (FDIC, 2009).[13] Ease in accessing such data varies from case to case. Data from public agencies and some commercial sources are sometimes readily accessible in publications, public-domain websites, and interactive interfaces designed to help users to locate information. Other relevant public health data are more difficult, and sometimes impossible, for a public health official to retrieve. Some difficulties are bureaucratic, such as procedural barriers imposed by agencies or companies that require paperwork, data-use agreements, payment of fees, account enrollments, or other special provisions to permit access. Some difficulties are related to quality and privacy concerns, as when agencies censor data they consider invalid because of small samples, or to the potential to disclose confidential information or personal identities. Some companies consider the information proprietary and refuse to release it out of concern that it will disclose intellectual property or yield crucial data to competitors.

Although proprietary concerns are a potential challenge to the sharing of private-sector data, the public today can already access much of this information readily on smart telephones, GPS devices, and Web browsers.

---

[13] "Unbanked" persons are considered financially vulnerable because the costs of using informal financial services, such as those of check-cashing businesses, are far greater than the costs of using mainstream financial institutions, such as banks (see, for example, FDIC, 2009).

BOX 2-2
Innovative Techniques and Queries for
Intersectoral Data-Gathering

- Google Searches—how many times users (in a given ZIP code) search for "flu" or "rash" or "poison" (used by GoogleFlu [Google, 2009]).
- Netherlands—primary-care data-monitoring sites (rotating sample of practices are compensated for daily or weekly input of patient and document data on symptoms, use rates, medications, and the like).
- Linkage of the Health Resources and Services Administration's Area Resource File and Bureau of Labor Statistics data by county and metropolitan and micropolitan statistical area to data provided by health departments.
- Monitoring of select data on alcohol sales and "driving under the influence" arrest frequency.
- Visit rates at local gyms.
- Sales of exercise equipment or by sporting goods chains.
- Funding of an "aggregator" agency (such as the Bureau of Economic Analysis, which collects data on the gross domestic product and national income and product accounts).
- Number of public health students in a county (data available from the Society for Public Health Education).

It is the government public health infrastructure that has not become "hardwired" into the wide array of data repositories. The government public health infrastructure needs tools and resources to use this wide array of data repositories. Data that many marketing firms access and use could be used to improve health. Innovative data-gathering techniques (see Box 2-2) will include partnering with other sectors. Building connections between public health, private data sources, and modeling enterprises would allow an evidence base to be built that, over time, will inform and empower decision-makers in influencing local social and environmental factors that strongly affect the health of communities.

In many cases, data are unavailable because a source agency or business has never been asked, does not view the sharing of such data as its responsibility, and has not invested any effort in organizing the information in ways that make it easy for others, particularly local community leaders, to retrieve it. That circumstance offers a potential opportunity for public health agency or community-organization outreach and collaboration with business. Making available data that can be used to build the evidence base and supporting appropriate local action and policies can give rise to logistical, resource, and proprietary challenges. To ease burdens on a source agency or company, such as clinical care providers that already have extensive administrative and reporting responsibilities, public health agencies and their partners must be thoughtful about the indicators requested. Requested data need to have a highly plausible relationship to health, and requests for more extensive or proprietary information should be avoided whenever possible. For example, local public health leaders may need to know only the number of fast-food restaurants in a community; industry sources may be glad to provide a regularly updated data set that includes the location of the restaurants but may oppose releasing data about ingredients and sales of individual products.

The HHS's CHDI described earlier has made valuable information available to users through a common platform—the HHS Data Warehouse (HHS, 2010a). Although openness and accessibility are two worthy ends, the committee noted that the initiative includes no intention to provide scientific direction or harmony to the world of indicators, to develop standards or unified guidance for those who use the HHS data, or to incorporate a forward-looking dimension to the initiative—one that gathers input from users and other information initiatives to feed into the evolution and continuous improvement of government data sets and elements to meet both the needs of the present and those of the future. When asked about the idea of direction or strategy, HHS staff associated with CHDI have explained that government data should go to users without any interpretation or modification (Park and Bilheimer, 2010). Although the committee understood the intent of that perspective—to allow exploration and innovation from many sources—it asserts that there is a vast difference between interpreting data with an eye toward advocating for a specific cause or policy and a kind of "translational" role of providing guidance on the use of data (for example, on the development and selection of indicators), on evolving needs for data, and on standards and methods for developing measures that can inform public health agencies and stakeholders working to improve population health. As discussed earlier, NCHS already receives the advice of two federal advisory committees, but their membership could be expanded to include representatives of other key government agencies (such as those in education, environment, and housing), more representatives of data users (including more public health officials or other practitioners), and researchers (including methodologists); likewise, their channels of communication with users, including policy analysts and decision-makers, could be enhanced to ensure an optimal level of end-user feedback.

CONCLUDING OBSERVATIONS

One of the persistent challenges to measuring health outcomes and one of the obstacles to any attempt to nurture standardization in the field is that many phenomena may be measured, but the field is much more advanced with respect to distal health outcomes (such as mortality and cancer incidence) and intermediate outcomes (or individual-level and behavioral determinants of health, such as smoking and obesity) than with respect to developing a knowledge base and valid, useful indicators of more upstream determinants of health (such as social cohesion, social support, the quality of housing, green spaces, and stress).

Although the determinants-of-health model is not formally understood by most members of the general public, people everywhere know what kind of community they would want to live in: one that is safe, with good schools, decent and affordable housing, access to healthful food, essential retail services, high-quality clinical care, and social and policy conditions that facilitate the financial and physical means to access all of these. Showing that some of the things people want can also improve their health is an important message in furthering the health of communities. Describing the evidence that links healthy communities to better health outcomes—that is, referring not to communities with healthy people but to communities that have the ingredients to support good health—must become part of the national and local narrative about health. Measurement provides the critical information for that narrative.

Measuring health-improvement processes and determinants with fidelity, understanding their relationship to the nation's well-being, and designing effective interventions all rest on harvesting information in a manner that is understandable, valid, timely, accurate, and integrated. The committee believes that measurement and reporting of information on health determinants and their associated outcomes can play an important role in galvanizing action by the myriad stakeholders that are in a position to influence population health.[14] The committee recognizes that measurement is a necessary but not sufficient ingredient for advancing population health. Other ingredients include addressing conflicting values, resource constraints, and a lack of political will at various levels of government and among stakeholders. Achieving population health will require a fundamental reconceptualization of health by the public and, similarly challenging, by decision-makers informed by coherent, relevant measures that can be monitored and acted on at the national, state, and local levels.

The committee has found that improved coordination and enhanced (for example, modernized) and new capacities are needed to strengthen the nation's population health statistics and information system. Federal statisti-

---

[14] Allocating a greater proportion of the US health dollar for population health would align national action with mounting evidence that socioecologic factors—the social and physical environment and government policies (protections, prohibitions, defaults, rewards, and incentives) that lead to particular levels of income, educational achievement, environmental exposure, and access to such necessities as nutritious food—have far greater effects on a nation's health than do actions at the individual level.

cal agencies, especially NCHS, have a central role to play, but collaboration and communication are needed among geographic levels and among sectors, given the wealth of information available in the private and nonprofit sectors that is often not integrated with government information to inform end users. The population health statistics and information system as a whole can play a more robust role in supporting the development of standardized indicator sets to demonstrate high-profile facts about the health of the nation, state, or community. However, the nation's population health statistics and information system will need revitalized leadership, including leadership by the nation's primary health statistics agency. That would require updating NCHS's mission to broaden its activities (going beyond improvement in its ability to perform its statutory duties to conducting more research on and interacting with users about, and providing scientific guidance pertinent to, its statistical work and translating NCHS and other data into indicators), enhancing the agency's capacities and ability to coordinate, as well as expanding its resources. Chapter 3 discusses in detail some solutions (including six recommendations) to the three sets of challenges just described.

REFERENCES

Academy Health. 2004. *Improving Federal Health Data for Coverage and Access Policy Development Needs.* Washington, DC: Academy Health.

AHRQ (Agency for Healthcare Research and Quality). 2007. *National Healthcare Disparities Report.* Rockville, MD: HHS.

BARHII (Bay Area Regional Health Inequities Initiative), and PHLP (Public Health Law & Policy). 2010. *Partners for Public Health: Working with Local, State, and Federal Agencies to Create Healthier Communities.* Oakland, CA: BARHII and PHLP.

Bilheimer, L. T. 2010. Evaluating metrics to improve population health. *Preventing Chronic Disease Public Health Research, Practice and Policy* 7(4). http://www.cdc.gov/pcd/issues/2010/jul/10_0016.htm (July 4, 2010).

Boufford, J. I., and P. R. Lee. 2001. *Health Policies for the 21st Century: Challenges and Recomendations for the U.S. Department of Health and Human Services.* New York: Milbank Memorial Fund.

Braveman, P., and S. Egerter. 2008. *Overcoming Obstacles to Health: Report from the Robert Wood Johnson Foundation to the Commission to Build a Healthier America.* Princeton, NJ: Robert Wood Johnson Foundation.

Braveman, P. A., C. Cubbin, S. Egerter, D. R. Williams, and E. Pamuk. 2010. Socioeconomic disparities in health in the United States: What the patterns tell us. *American Journal of Public Health* 100:S186-S196.

Brownson, R. C., R. Seiler, and A. A. Eyler. 2010. Measuring the impact of pulic helath policy. *Preventing Chronic Disease Public Health Research, Practice and Policy* 7(4). http://www.cdc.gov/pcd/issues/2010/jul/09_0249.htm (July 4, 2010).

Burd-Sharpe, S., K. Lewis, E. Borges Martins, A. Sen, and W. H. Draper. 2010. *The Measure of America: American Human Development Report, 2008-2009.* Brooklyn, NY: Columbia University Press.

CDC (Centers for Disease Control and Prevention). 2010. *Series of Reports from the National Health Interview Survey.* http://www.cdc.gov/nchs/nhis/nhis_series.htm (November 15, 2010).

Commonwealth Fund. 2009. *The Path to a High Performance US Health System: A 2020 Vision and the Policies to Pave the Way.* New York: Commonwealth Fund.

Community Health Status Indicators. 2009. *Community Health Status Indicators Project Fact Sheet.* Washington, DC: HHS.

County Health Rankings. 2010. *Updated Model: Background.* http://www.countyhealth rankings.org/print/about-project/background (February 17, 2010).

Department of Health, Education, and Welfare. 1969. *Toward a Social Report.* Washington, DC: Government Printing Office.

Donabedian, A. 1988. The quality of care: How can it be assessed? *Journal of the American Medical Association* 260(12):1743-1748.

Egerter, S., P. Braveman, T. Sadegh-Nobari, R. Grossman-Kahn, and M. Dekker. 2009. *Education Matters for Health, Issue Brief 6: Education and Health.* Princeton, NJ: Robert Wood Johnson Foundation.

Executive Office of the President. 2009. *Transparency and Open Government.* http://www.whitehouse.gov/the_press_office/TransparencyandOpenGovernment (October 25, 2010).

FDIC (Federal Deposit Insurance Corporation). 2009. *Financial education and the future: The banking industry's role in helping consumers manage money and build assets.* Washington, DC: FDIC.

Federal Interagency Forum on Child and Family Statistics. 2010. *America's Children in Brief: Key National Indicators of Well-being, 2010.* Washington, DC: Government Printing Office.

Friedman, D. J., and R. G. Parrish. 2009a. Is community health assessment worthwhile? *Journal of Public Health Management & Practice* 15(1):3-9.

Friedman, D. J., and R. G. Parrish. 2009b. *Phase I: Report to the National Committee on Vital and Health Statistics, Reconsidering Shaping a Health Statistics Vision for the 21st Century.* Washington, DC: HHS.

Friedman, D. J., E. L. Hunter, and G. R. Parrish II, eds. 2005. *Health Statistics: Shaping Policy and Practice to Improve the Population's Health.* New York: Oxford University Press.

Gallup–Healthways. 2008. *The U.S. Well-being Index.* http://www.well-beingindex.com/methodology.asp (September 8, 2010).

GAO (Government Accountability Office). 2004. *Informing Our Nation: Improving How to Understand and Access the USA's Position and Progress—Report to the Chairman, Subcommittee on Science, Technology, and Space, Committee on Commerce, Science, and Transportation, U.S. Senate.* Washington, DC: GAO.

Goff, D. C., Jr., L. Brass, L. T. Braun, J. B. Croft, J. D. Flesch, F. G. R. Fowkes, Y. Hong, V. Howard, S. Huston, S. F. Jencks, R. Luepker, T. Manolio, C. O'Donnell, R. Marie Robertson, W. Rosamond, J. Rumsfeld, S. Sidney, and Z. J. Zheng. 2007a. Essential features of a surveillance system to support the prevention and management of heart disease and stroke: A scientific statement from the American Heart Association councils on epidemiology and prevention, stroke, and cardiovascular nursing and the interdisciplinary working groups on quality of care and outcomes research and atherosclerotic peripheral vascular disease. *Circulation* 115(1):127-155.

Goff, D. C., Jr., H. C. Gerstein, H. N. Ginsberg, W. C. Cushman, K. L. Margolis, R. P. Byington, J. B. Buse, S. Genuth, J. L. Probstfield, and D. G. Simons-Morton. 2007b. Prevention of cardiovascular disease in persons with Type 2 Diabetes Mellitus: Current knowledge and rationale for the action to control cardiovascular risk in diabetes (ACCORD) trial. *The American Journal of Cardiology* 99(12, Suppl 1):S4-S20.

Google. 2009. *Google: Flu Trends.* http://www.google.org/flutrends/about/how.html (October 25, 2010).

Healthcare Cost and Utilization Project. 2010. *HCUP Partners Healthcare Cost and Utilization Project.* http://www.hcup-us.ahrq.gov/partners.jsp (September 28, 2010).

HHS (Department of Health and Human Services). 2009. *Healthy People 2020: The Road Ahead*. http://www.healthypeople.gov/hp2020 (October 2, 2009).

HHS. 2010a. *Community Health Data Initiative*. http://www.hhs.gov/open/plan/opengovernmentplan/initiatives/initiative.html (August 19, 2010).

HHS. 2010b. *Community Health Data Initiative: Data Sets*. http://www.hhs.gov/open/datasets/index.html (October 25, 2010).

HHS. 2010c. *Healthy People 2010: What Are the Leading Health Indicators?* http://www.healthypeople.gov/lhi/lhiwhat.htm (October 25, 2010).

HHS. 2010d. *HHS Gateway to Data and Statistics*. http://www.hhs-stat.net (November 15, 2010).

HHS, CDC, and NCVHS (National Committee on Vital and Health Statistics). 2002. *Shaping a Health Statistics Vision for the 21st Century*. Washington, DC: HHS.

IOM (Institute of Medicine). 2008. *State of the USA Health Indicators: Letter Report*. Washington, DC: The National Academies Press.

IOM. 2010a. *Leading Health Indicators for Healthy People 2020*. http://www8.nationalacademies.org/cp/committeeview.aspx?key=49269 (October 25, 2010).

IOM. 2010b. Transcript, *Second Meeting of the IOM Committee on Public Health Strategies to Improve Health*. Washington, DC: IOM.

Kindig, D. A., Y. Asada, and B. Booske. 2008. A population health framework for setting national and state health goals. *Journal of the American Medical Association* 299(17):2081-2083.

Krieger, J., and D. L. Higgins. 2002. Housing and health: Time again for public health action. *American Journal of Public Health* 92(5):758-768.

Lahelma, E., P. Martikainen, M. Laaksonen, and A. Aittomäki. 2004. Pathways between socioeconomic determinants of health. *Journal of Epidemiology and Community Health* 58(4):327-332.

Lalonde, M. 1981. *A New Perspective on the Health of Canadians: A Working Document*. Ottowa, Canada: Ministry of National Health and Welfare.

Luck, J., C. Chang, E. R. Brown, and J. Lumpkin. 2006. Using local health information to promote public health. *Health Affairs* 25(4):979-991.

Lumpkin, J. R., and M. S. Richards. 2002. Transforming the public health information infrastructure. *Health Affairs* 21(6):45-56.

The Marmot Review. 2010. *Fair Society, Healthy Lives: Strategic Review of Health Inequalities in England Post 2010*. London, England: The Marmot Review.

McGinnis, J. M., and W. H. Foege. 1993. Actual causes of death in the United States. *Journal of the American Medical Association* 270(18):2007-2012.

Mendez-Luck, C. A., H. Yu, Y. Y. Meng, M. Jhawar, and S. P. Wallace. 2007. Estimating health conditions for small areas: Asthma symptom prevalence for state legislative districts. *Health Services Research* 42(6 Pt 2):2389-2409.

Mikkonen, J., and D. Raphael. 2010. *Social Determinants of Health: The Canadian Facts*. Toronto, Canada: York University School of Health Policy and Management.

Miringoff, M., and M. L. Miringoff. 1999. *The Social Health of the Nation: How America Is Really Doing*. New York: Oxford University Press.

Mokdad, A. H., J. S. Marks, D. F. Stroup, and J. L. Gerberding. 2004. Actual causes of death in the United States, 2000. *Journal of the American Medical Association* 291(10):1238-1245.

National Program of Cancer Registries. 2010. *NPCR: About the Program*. http://www.cdc.gov/cancer/npcr/about.htm (September 28, 2010).

NCHS (National Center for Health Statistics). 1998. *Health, United States, 1998: With Socioeconomic Status and Health Chartbook*. Hyattsville, MD: HHS.

NCHS. 2008. *Final Report of the National Health Interview Survey Review Panel to the NCHS Board of Scientific Counselors: Executive Summary*. Atlanta, GA: CDC.

NCHS. 2009. *Report of the NHANES Review Panel to the NCHS Board of Scientific Counselors.* Atlanta, GA: CDC.

NCVHS (National Committee for Vital and Health Statistics). 2010. *Toward Enhanced Information Capacities for Health: An NCVHS Concept Paper.* Washington, DC: HHS.

NRC (National Research Council). 2009. *Principles and Practices for a Federal Statistical Agency.* 4th Edition. Washington, DC: The National Academies Press.

O'Grady. 2006. Commentary-improving federal health data: The essential partnership between researcher and policy maker. *Health Services Research* 41(3):984-989.

Park, T., and L. Bilheimer. 2010 (May 18). *HHS Community Health Data Initiative.* Presentation to the IOM Committee on Public Health Strategies to Improve Health. Washington, DC: IOM.

Parrish, R. G. 2010. Measuring population health outcomes. *Preventing Chronic Disease Public Health Research, Practice and Policy* 7(4). http://www.cdc.gov/pcd/issues/2010/jul/10_0005.htm (July 4, 2010).

Population Association of America. 2010. *Population Association of America.* http://www.populationassociation.org (September 8, 2010).

Public Health Institute. 2010. *Data Sets, Data Platforms, Data Utility: Resource Compendium.* Oakland, CA: Public Health Institute.

Robert Wood Johnson Foundation Commission to Build a Healthier America. 2009. *Beyond Health Care: New Directions to a Healthier America: Recommendations from the Robert Wood Johnson Foundation Commission to Build a Healthier America.* Princeton, NJ: Robert Wood Johnson Foundation.

Rothwell, C. J., E. J. Sondik, and B. Guyer. 2004. A delay in publication of the "annual summary of vital statistics" and the need for new vital registration and statistics systems for the United States. *Pediatrics* 114(6):1671-1672.

Rudolph, L. 2009 (December). *Healthy Communities.* Presented to UC Berkeley Policy Roundtable—Center for Cities and Schools. Berkeley, CA: UC Berkeley.

Safran, C., M. Bloomrosen, W. Hammond, S. Labkoff, S. Markel-Fox, P. C. Tang, D. E. Detmer, and with input from the expert panel. 2007. Toward a national framework for the secondary use of health data: An American Medical Informatics Association white paper. *Journal of the American Medical Informatics Association* 14(1):1-9.

Schwab, K., X. Sala-i-Martin, and R. Greenhill. 2010. *The Global Competitiveness Report 2010-2011.* Geneva, Switzerland: World Economic Forum.

Schwartz, S. 2008. *The United States Vital Statistics System: The Role of State and Local Health Departments.* New York, NY: United Nations.

Seattle and King County Public Health Department. 2010. *King County Community Health Indicators.* http://www.kingcounty.gov/healthservices/health/data/chi.aspx (January 6, 2010).

Secretary's Advisory Committee on National Health Promotion and Disease Prevention Objectives for 2020. 2010. *Healthy People 2020: An Opportunity to Address Societal Determinants of Health in the U.S.* Washington, DC: HHS.

Starr, P., and S. Starr. 1995. Reinventing vital statistics. The impact of changes in information technology, welfare policy, and health care. *Public Health Reports* 110(5):534-544.

Summers, C., L. Cohen, A. Havusha, F. Sliger, and T. Farley. 2009. *Take care New York 2012: A policy for a healthier New York City.* New York, NY: New York City Department of Health and Mental Hygiene.

SUSA (State of the USA). 2010. *The State of the USA.* http://www.stateoftheusa.org (September 1, 2010).

Trust for America's Health. 2010. *State Data.* http://healthyamericans.org/states (October 15, 2010).

University of Wisconsin Population Health Institute. 2010. *Mobilizing Action Toward Community Health (MATCH): Population Health Metrics, Solid Partnerships, and Real Incentives*. http://uwphi.pophealth.wisc.edu/pha/match.htm (June 10, 2010).

Ver Ploeg, M., V. Breneman, T. Farrigan, K. Hamrick, D. Hopkins, P. Kaufman, B. H. Lin, M. Nord, T. Smith, R. Williams, K. Kinnson, C. Olander, A. Singh, and E. Tuckermanty. 2009. *Access to affordable nutritious food: Measuring and understanding food deserts and their consequences—report to congress*. Washington, DC: Department of Agriculture.

Virginia Commonwealth University. 2009. *Center on Human Needs*. http://www.humanneeds.vcu.edu (August 5, 2010).

Wold, C. 2008. *Health Indicators: A Review of Reports Currently in Use*. Conducted for The State of the USA. Wold and Associates.

3

Measuring Health for Improved Decisions and Performance

In this chapter, the committee presents six recommendations to address the challenges described in Chapter 2: (1) improving coordination at the national level, beginning with the primary federal health statistics agency (the National Center for Health Statistics [NCHS]) and with federal health data and statistics activities in general[1]; (2) adopting the determinants of health perspective at a fundamental level (to complement the health system's predominantly biomedical orientation); and (3) enhancing responsiveness of the population health information system to the needs of end users.

IMPROVING COORDINATION AT THE NATIONAL LEVEL

Critical to progress on these challenges is leadership at the federal level, largely by Department of Health and Human Services (HHS). While HHS has 30 statistical offices and programs, NCHS, which is located within the Centers for Disease Control and Prevention, is the nation's lead health-statistics agency (NRC, 2009). Although the array of information produced by those multiple efforts is rich, its great fragmentation—and overlap, suboptimal coordination, and remaining unaddressed gaps (for example, in data elements and in research needed to improve the quality, usefulness,

---

[1] The HHS Data Council plays a key role in facilitating intradepartmental coordination on data and statistics issues. The Council has supported the development of the HHS Gateway to Data and Statistics (HHS, 2010), which represents one of several HHS efforts to make federal health data more available and accessible. The Council's role in coordinating HHS data systems has also been discussed at a meeting of the Secretary's Advisory Committee on National Health Promotion and Disease Prevention Objectives for 2020 (HHS, 2009b).

and breadth of the information available)—makes the utility of the system's combined efforts less than it should be.

Many of the data sets described in Chapter 2 are built from core data elements that have been static for many years and reflect the sum of the health of individuals with few data on measures of the health of a community. The committee's vision of measurement includes both a reconsideration of the use of older measures that may be less amenable to local action and accountability and the building of new measures and potentially new measurement systems that report on more recently recognized loci for intervention.

NCHS's current mission is "to provide statistical information that will guide actions and policies to improve the health of the American people. As the Nation's principal health statistics agency, NCHS leads the way with accurate, relevant, and timely data" (CDC, 2009). Although recognizing the statutory underpinnings of its mission, the committee believes that the current implementation of the NCHS mission is too limited (e.g., to conducting surveys). The 2002 HHS document *Developing a 21st Century Vision for Health Statistics* states that the NCHS vision should (HHS, 2002)

- Reflect all manifestations of health and health care delivery.
- Encompass population health, transactions between the population and the health care delivery system, and the health care delivery system.
- Address the relationship and potential synergy between public and private health data sets and national, state, and locally maintained data.

Those three points are congruent with the committee's findings about the statistics and information system's needs, gaps, and opportunities. NCHS's current mission statement and the committee's understanding of the agency's scope of work suggest that its current role consists primarily of conducting several major surveys on population health, as well as managing the nation's vital statistics system and managing surveys of nursing homes, hospitals, outpatient facilities, and other clinical care providers (NRC, 2009). The committee believes that NCHS can and should play a broader leadership role in the population health information system, expanding its analytic capabilities, its research activities, its ability to collaborate with those who use its data, and its ability to help to modernize and integrate the system. Transforming the way the mission of NCHS is implemented could broaden the array of activities in which NCHS engages beyond surveys and basic statistical work and toward activities that facilitate and provide guidance for the "translation" of data into information and knowledge that decision-makers and communities can use.

Facilitating a more highly integrated data system and a national population health measurement strategy requires both governance and a high level of scientific guidance. In this chapter, the committee believes that NCHS, as the lead national health-statistics agency, must be strengthened to improve its ability to lead a system-wide effort toward better coordination and, as discussed below, enhanced information capacities for the health system. It is important to note here the roles of two federal advisory committees affiliated with NCHS: the Board of Scientific Counselors, which provides advice to NCHS, and the National Committee on Vital and Health Statistics (NCVHS), which is chartered to advise the secretary of HHS but is staffed in NCHS and closely identified with its work. NCVHS also has a population health subcommittee.[2]

The committee recognizes that two provisions of the Affordable Care Act (ACA)[3] have potential pertinence to strengthening the nation's population health information system. First, and most important, the new National Prevention, Health Promotion, and Public Health Council (NPHPPHC)— comprised of twelve cabinet secretaries and agency heads, under the leadership of the Surgeon General (Public Law 111-148)—offers an unprecedented opportunity for all sectors of government to come together around a de facto Health in All Policies effort. In recent years, there have been efforts around the country to examine the ramifications of all types of policy decisions on health outcomes, by using such tools as health impact assessments, as part of an approach called Health in All Policies, which calls for considering the health effects of all government policies and is internationally used (for example, in the European Union) (CDC, 2010b; Koivusalo, 2010). The council is to make "recommendations to the President and the Congress concerning the most pressing health issues confronting the United States and changes in Federal policy to achieve national wellness, health promotion, and public health goals, including the reduction of tobacco use, sedentary behavior, and poor nutrition" (Congressional Research Service, 2010).

The executive order establishing the council creates a forum for collaboration and coordination among twelve federal departments and agencies that have roles with implications for population health. For the purposes of enhancing the nation's population health information system, the council's composition (for example, the inclusion of other agencies) could provide an independent or fresh perspective from outside HHS that could be useful in supporting the department and NCHS (in addition to ensuring that the transformation of NCHS takes place as a primary requirement for meeting

---

[2] The Subcommittee focuses on both "(1) population-based data such as vital statistics and health surveys concerning the U.S. population generally and (2) data about specific vulnerable groups within the population which are disadvantaged by virtue of their special health needs, economic status, race and ethnicity, disability, age, or area of residence" (NCVHS, 2008).

[3] The Patient Protection and Affordable Care Act and the Health Care and Education Affordability Reconciliation Act, known jointly as the Affordable Care Act (ACA).

the nation's population health information needs). The council's work could have ramifications for cross-department information and data efforts. For example, as discussed in Chapter 2 and below, data on determinants of health reside in many government agencies outside HHS, and linkages to make such data available to the public health community are not optimally developed or are in very early stages of development (the US Department of Agriculture *Food Environment Atlas* is an exception; see USDA, 2010). The council, under the leadership of the surgeon general, has been charged with preparing a national prevention strategy and an annual report on its progress in implementing the strategy.

Second, the act includes a provision to establish a Key National Indicators Initiative (Congressional Research Service, 2010). The initiative will develop and disseminate key indicators on health, education, the economy, agriculture, transportation, and other parts of American society in recognition of the cross-cutting information needs involved in forming a full picture of the status of American society. With respect to health, it could create a forum for integrating data from different levels of government and sectors.

A stronger and adequately resourced NCHS would be in a position to play a coordinating and leadership role in rationalizing, harmonizing, and integrating population health data collection, analysis, and reporting efforts and to provide scientific guidance on developing and selecting indicators and reflecting on the effects of various determinants of health. In continually reviewing the nation's population health information system and its contributions to understanding health at the community and subpopulation level, NCHS could facilitate a move toward a more coherent system. In reviewing the major domains in which data are collected, the agency could call for new indicators to be added and for those of decreasing relevance to be culled. The process could be likened to those in other important societal arenas, such as changing the components of the consumer price index or the stocks included in the Dow Jones Industrial Average.

In its 2009 report *Principles and Practices for a Federal Statistical Agency* (Fourth Edition), the National Research Council's Committee on National Statistics outlined the key characteristics and roles for such agencies as NCHS, including Practice 8 (an active research program intended to improve data content and the design and operation of data collection and to make information more useful to decision-makers) and Practice 11 (coordination and cooperation with other statistical agencies) (NRC, 2009). As noted in Chapter 2, two recent external reviews of NCHS's National Health Interview Survey (NHIS) and its National Health and Nutrition Examination Survey have found that the agency needs greater financial and staff resources to undertake improvements in these major statistical activities, including methodologic and other research (NCHS, 2008, 2009). Three-fourths of NCHS's estimated budget supports the purchase of data collection and reporting services from state and local governments, the Bureau of the Census, and private contractors (NRC, 2009), leaving few resources to support those other critical endeavors.

The committee has learned that others have examined the nation's health statistics and information system and have suggested ways to enhance coordination and integration to serve the overarching objective of improving population health. Proposals have included a call, in the 2002 HHS document *Shaping a Health Statistics Vision for the 21st Century,* for an "integrating hub" to facilitate coordination of statistical activities within HHS (HHS et al., 2002) and a call for a population health record (Friedman and Parrish, 2010).

In its information-gathering sessions, the committee learned from public health practitioners that they often lack local-level data needed for fundamental planning and priority-setting and that federally produced statistics or measures meet only some of their information needs (IOM, 2010a,b). The committee heard repeatedly that the federal government's own efforts to collect health-related data have historically occurred in silos (e.g., along vertical programmatic lines, with little or insufficient cross-cutting integration and collaboration) both within HHS and with other government departments and agencies. The population health information system as a whole is not ideally structured to facilitate interaction, collaboration, and data exchange and integration between the public and private sectors.

Another concern is minimizing inefficiencies to avoid burdensome procedures and costs for agencies and organizations, such as requests to provide the same data in different formats to different national, state, or local entities. Coordination is necessary to facilitate user access to data that originate from different government sources. That suggests the need for coordination to establish systems that maximize efficiency, streamline bureaucratic procedures, and expand the new HHS data warehouse (through the Community Health Data Initiative [CHDI] effort) while facilitating the integration of data from different sources on population health into an accessible, well-designed, and interactive interface to enable users to obtain relevant data at the geographic level of interest easily (see Chapter 2 and Appendix B discussion of CHDI, which represents a start).

Given the challenging nature of coordination and integration and the centrality of the need, the committee believes that a patchwork approach will not be adequate to meet the information needs of the health system. Comprehensive change, beginning at the core of federal work in this field, is needed to lead the way in addressing the gaps discussed in Chapter 2 and to support the development of a population health information system capable of responding to and forecasting the opportunities and meeting the challenges of the next decade and beyond.

Recommendation 1

The committee recommends that:

1. The Secretary of Health and Human Services transform the mission of the National Center for Health Statistics to provide leadership to a renewed population health information system through enhanced coordination, new capacities, and better integration of the determinants of health.
2. The National Prevention, Health Promotion, and Public Health Council include in its annual report to Congress on its national prevention and health-promotion strategy an update on the progress of the National Center for Health Statistics transformation.

The committee believes that NCHS is the right body to provide leadership in changing the nation's population health information system because it is the nation's main health-statistics entity, has a long history of work and accomplishment, and has many of the requisite connections with other federal agencies. Although federal agencies depend to a large extent on political realities and therefore have some limitations of independence, the committee was not able to envision a sustainable source of funding that would support a new public–private entity charged with playing the major coordinating role that it has described. The committee believes that the reporting structure laid out below, which includes an accountability mechanism, could help to buffer the agency against political vicissitudes that may affect its evolution to greater strength and capability.

The transformation of NCHS will require changes in the agency's mission (or, more specifically, its implementation), capabilities, authority, and resources. Its current output is largely statistically analyzed data, but as described in this chapter, its role needs to be broadened to include capacities and activities to translate data into information and to conduct related research, such as research on the development and construction of indicators. Although "analysis by a statistical agency does not advocate policies or take partisan positions" (NRC, 2009), the committee believes that there is a substantial difference between advocacy and playing an active and central role in improving the quality and usefulness of indicators and other tools for disseminating population health information and enhancing the research infrastructure and agenda to support these activities.

An independent and influential external body will be necessary to oversee the progress of the transformation. Given the cross-cutting nature of the new NPHPPHC and the fundamental value and necessity of population health information for the prevention and health-promotion strategy that it is charged to develop, the committee believes that the council (with input from their Advisory Group on Prevention, Health Promotion, and Integrative and Public Health, which can provide input from other sectors) can play an important role in monitoring changes in NCHS that can support or facilitate improvements in the nation's population health information system as a whole. A considerable challenge is that NCHS will require continuing funding outside the political process. Although statistical agencies, such as NCHS, do not advocate, some of the information they produce could suggest or lead to action that is not consonant with particular political agendas. A possible solution would be to devote a portion of HHS funds to NCHS without requiring yearly appropriations.

The national prevention and health-promotion strategy is intended to include specific goals, and the NPHPPHC is asked to describe "corrective actions recommended by the Council and actions taken by relevant agencies and organizations to meet" the goals.[4] The committee believes that NCVHS, working at the behest of the secretary of HHS, may serve as a technical resource to the NPHPPHC in evaluating the success of NCHS's transformation (and the NCVHS Subcommittee on Population Health has additional expertise that would lend itself to this task, although it would need to include public health practice and community development). Although the executive order establishing the council does not explicitly refer to the centrality of statistics and measurement (and this is not one of the kinds of expertise listed in the charter of the advisory group of the council, which is still under development), the committee notes that the council's first annual report lists eight principles that guide its work, including reviewing "data on the leading and underlying causes of death" as part of its focus on prevention (National Prevention Health Promotion and Public Health Council, 2010).

An adequately resourced and transformed NCHS would possess the mission, capabilities, resources, and authority to improve aspects of current activities and to undertake new activities. NCHS could

- Coordinate research on and support the development of—within HHS and in collaboration with relevant stakeholders—several population health information tools and processes described in recommendations elsewhere in this chapter:
  - A standardized set of measures of community health (see Recommendation 2).
  - A standardized set of health-outcome indicators that can be used at the national, state, and local levels (see Recommendation 2).
  - A summary measure of population health (see Recommendation 2).
  - Modeling to elucidate the complex relationships between health and its determinants (see Recommendation 6).

---

[4] Executive Order No. 13544, 75 Fed. Reg. 33983 (June 10, 2010). http://edocket.access.gpo.gov/2010/pdf/2010-14613.pdf (accessed June 14, 2010).

- Modernize national data sets to concentrate on indicators known to be pertinent to many conditions (for example, by combining NHIS, the Behavioral Risk Factor Surveillance System, and other questions about important social and environmental determinants not currently tracked in the data sets) and focus less on specific disease data sets.
- Make recommendations about modern survey methods to collect more valid data efficiently. Modernizing could include better ways of performing household surveys, collecting responses electronically, and maximizing opportunities afforded by the shift from landline telephones to mobile phones.
- Provide leadership in the uniform application of novel analytic tools.
- Collaborate with other health-related government agencies, including on the collection of (and acting on) information on their user experience, their needs, and their use of available statistics.

NCHS already has strong or growing collaborative relationships with an array of federal departments and agencies, such as the Bureau of the Census and various HHS agencies and statistical units. NCHS could strengthen or cultivate additional linkages with other federal departments that produce statistics and information relevant to population health—such as the Departments of Agriculture, Transportation, Labor, and Education—and with external (private-sector) data organizations.

The committee acknowledges that calling for strengthening of a government agency does not address the fundamental need for coordination among public- and private-sector data sources. However, it is pleased to note (and endorses) the NPHPPHC's guiding principle pertaining to public–private collaboration (National Prevention Health Promotion and Public Health Council, 2010), and believes that a federal advisory committee like NCVHS (which includes private-sector representatives, whose numbers could be expanded) can play a role in facilitating interactions between, for example, government and business.

Bringing Coherence to Indicators

Building an understanding of the forces that shape and create health requires development and testing of new and evolving indicators and continuing tests of their relationships to one another—for example, as facilitated by modeling. On the pages that follow, the committee describes indicators that are inadequately developed (community-health indicators), require rationalization and standardization (health-outcome indicators for national, state, and local data sets), or are in evolution (summary measures of population health).

A Standard Set of Community-Health Indicators

Chapter 2 summarized recent efforts to measure the health of communities and present the results as a ranking or in comparative fashion (Communities Count, 2008; Community Health Status Indicators, 2009; County Health Rankings, 2010; Saskatoon Regional Health Authority, 2007). Most of the indicators produced by such efforts are aggregations of various health and risk measures of individuals at specific times rather than measures of the overall health of communities in and of themselves (i.e., the health of the social and physical environments in a community). The current usage of the term *community health indicators* differs somewhat from the committee's thinking about true measures of community health that convey information about characteristics of the community as opposed to aggregated data on its individual members.

Community-health indicators pertain largely to the local level. Consensus on the appropriate domains and indicators at this time is either impossible or extremely challenging. For example, there are different measures of "walkability" in a community—some that have been used in studies, such as pedestrian facilities (for example, sidewalk completeness and traffic-signal density) and street connectivity (street and intersection density), and some that have been included in municipal or community reports (for example, the ratio of sidewalks to roads in a community and the distance to such amenities as grocery stores, libraries, and parks; see, for example, Jakubowski and Frumkin, 2010; Zhu and Lee, 2008). Similarly, for healthy-food access or availability, there is no consensus about what indicators are best for different purposes—whether to select the ratio of convenience stores to grocery stores, the prevalence of fast-food outlets, or some other metric—and indicator validation has only recently begun (Glanz, 2009; Lytle, 2009). Social cohesion, trust, and support; health literacy; social vibrancy; and different types of environments all require consensus with respect to specific indicators (Lantz and Pritchard, 2010) that could be used and tested to further develop a balanced portfolio of community-health indicators. There also is no high-quality, widely accepted overarching measure of environmental health from an exposure perspective, although there are several focused measures, such as ozone and $PM_{2.5}$ (Jakubowski and Frumkin, 2010). Both a more robust set of indicators and a set of criteria for selecting among them are needed (as an example, see Healthy People 2020 [HP 2020] criteria for selecting objectives [HHS, 2009a]).

Beyond their direct effects on the health of individuals, social, environmental, and economic factors rooted in communities also influence the overall health of communities, which in turn influences the health of individuals. (Chapter 1 summarizes some of the evidence on the determinants of health.) Community-health indicators are needed to capture, understand, and describe those factors to community members and to decision-makers.

Domains that require representation include aspects of the physical environment (such as sidewalks, pollution, green space, and housing), of social support (such as cohesion, social capital, and social efficacy and engagement), and of community vibrancy (such as participation in the arts and sports). The literature exploring the use of those indicators is developing. Some of the domains that may serve as examples include

- Income and income distribution, education, unemployment and job security, employment and working conditions, early-childhood development, food insecurity, housing, social exclusion, social-safety network, sex, and race (Mikkonen and Raphael, 2010).
- Scope of early-childhood development programs, education and skills, employment and good jobs, minimum income for healthy living, and healthy communities (community capital) (The Marmot Review, 2010).
- Food and water, housing, a nonhazardous work environment, a nonhazardous physical environment, security in childhood, important primary relationships, economic security, physical security, and education (Doyle and Gough, 1991).

To track and understand those domains, public health agencies and their health-system partners at state and local levels require data from other sectors. For example, a local public health agency may have access to some indicators of the social determinants of health, such as educational attainment and income, but not to others, including more complex (or less well-understood or well-defined) community features or resources, such as social capital (Drukker et al., 2005; Prentice, 2006), the availability of healthy and fresh foods in the community, or the health literacy of its inhabitants. An employer or school planning department may need data on the community's use of public recreational venues, such as parks, in developing physical-activity interventions.

The presence of smoking restrictions, requirements of menu labeling (before the ACA provision that pre-empted such local and state laws), pedistrian-friendly planning, and effective regulation of the clinical care system are all examples of regulatory and enforcement environments as good markers of aspects of community health (e.g., National Complete Streets Coalition, 2010).[5] Communities that have higher levels of civic engagement

---

[5] One example of a potential area for legislative attention pertaining to the built environment is found in the work of the National Complete Streets Coalition. The coalition is a diverse partnership advocating for national, state, and local legislative action to institute "complete street" policies (e.g., policies that influence transportation planning and seek to ensure that transportation in all communities is optimally safe, results in lower emissions, and facilitates increased physical activity) (National Complete Streets Coalition, 2010).

and similar characteristics are typically better equipped than others to enact policies that change environmental conditions to foster healthier behaviors (such as access to healthy foods and places for physical activity). Access to supermarkets and healthy food sources (and, conversely, the density of fast-food outlets, convenience stores, and liquor stores) is of established relevance to overweight and obesity and thus points to potentially important indicators of community health that could be routinely collected and shared.

In summary, although a number of national indicator sets include a few indicators of broad social determinants of health, the committee believes that unified guidance is needed to describe and build an evidence base for an actionable set of additional indicators that would support community decision-making with respect to local health-promoting initiatives. Data availability and research elucidating causal pathways may pose limitations, and the committee believes that galvanizing local partners to work in concert toward health gains will require a shared understanding of the factors that influence the health of communities. Developing that understanding rests on capturing new indicators and exploring their utility through experimental and observational studies and modeling.

The committee finds that many of the so-called community indicators that are in use focus largely on aggregates of individuals' social risk factors, such as income and education, such health outcomes as mortality and disease-specific morbidity rates, and such individual risk factors as smoking. The committee recognizes that the evidence base available in many of the categories discussed here, including geographic relevance, is underdeveloped. It believes that knowing and communicating about the health of communities is essential for informing health-improvement efforts. Small area (community level) analysis is critical to identifying disparities, such as vulnerable subpopulations with considerably poorer health outcomes than those of the larger population (e.g., a metropolitan statistical area) within which they are embedded. The committee acknowledges the need for resources in capturing new information and understanding it.

A Standard Set of Health-Outcome Indicators

As discussed in Chapter 2, indicators of population health in the United States currently form a rich amalgam rather than a coherent whole that can be used in public health practice in a way that is considered and consistent over time. Although several existing measurement efforts described in Chapter 2 include a variety of health outcomes (i.e., distal outcomes such as disease rates and disease-specific mortality rates), and although such indicators are sometimes similar from one set to another and based on similar or identical sources of data, no standardized set of indicators has been vetted and found to be useful in serving population health planning at all levels.

The many sets of health indicators currently in use arose, understandably, to meet users' varied needs. However, the existence of many indicator sets precludes gaining a single, coherent picture of population health in a consistent manner among communities and regions. Similarly, federal data sets and state and local efforts are not coordinated to the fullest extent to ensure efficiency and completeness, usefulness, and timeliness of the data. That can limit the ability of data-collection efforts to add relevant new indicators as the science develops and to discard indicators that are no longer useful. The committee believes that developing a core set of health-outcome indicators that identify priority health outcomes (aggregate distal individual health outcomes and indicators of behavioral risk) is a necessary step in a broader process to improve coordination and local-to-national relevance of data collection and indicator reporting efforts; however, such a set would not meet all needs, and it would need to evolve.

Indicators of health outcomes pertain to all geographic levels and refer to distal outcomes, such as disease and death. Such indicators are currently found in indicator sets like those described above. A core standardized set of indicators would ideally reflect a convergence of national, state, and local priorities, preferably embedded in a major national initiative, such as HP 2020 or the Key National Indicators Initiative. It would facilitate "apples to apples" comparisons of jurisdictions, allow the aggregation of local data to yield national figures, and support the linkage of national objectives, such as those in the Healthy People effort, to state and local objectives.

Summary Measures of Population Health

Because a summary measure of population health, described in detail below, would serve as a marker of the progress of the nation and its communities in improving health, it is important that it be implemented in data-collection and public communication efforts at the federal, state, and local levels. The committee believes that public officials need to take steps to educate Americans about the meaning of summary measures of population health and their linkage to determinants that are amenable to action at individual and societal levels.

Summary measures of population health that integrate information about mortality and morbidity are distal-outcomes measures that permit public health professionals, academicians, and decision-makers to understand trends in the health of populations and subpopulations. Referred to also as health-adjusted life years (HALYs), these measures have been used in local public health practice (Kominski et al., 2002) and in international settings (Ferrer et al., 2002; McIntosh et al., 2009; Murray et al., 2002) to establish distributions and burdens of disease, and they are routinely used in other nations to inform resource-allocation priorities in public health and clinical care (for an Australian example, see Mitchell et al., 2009; for a British example, see Pearson and Rawlins, 2005; for an overview of use in other countries, see Neumann and Greenberg, 2009). Despite continuing development and validation by US and foreign academicians of the health-related quality-of-life measures on which HALYs are built, US health professionals and decision-makers have been slow to adopt them (Fryback et al., 2007).

In the United States and internationally, mortality-based indicators have functioned as the predominant final-outcome measure of the health of populations. Life expectancy and death rates provide important information about the different experience of nations, communities, and subpopulations. Disaggregated and presented by region and sociodemographic characteristic, they furnish critical information about health status and health inequalities that can be readily understood by decision-makers and members of the public. However, life expectancy is a blunt tool. It cannot capture the diminution in life experience and capacities that is associated with the chronic illnesses and injuries that are of increasing prevalence in modern society. Lessening of the burden of disease and attendant improvement in health-related quality of life are important objectives of population-based and clinical care delivery interventions. For example, use of life expectancy does not capture any information about the gains associated with the better dentition that accompanies fluoridated water or the better vision achieved with cataract surgery, and it only incompletely captures the effects of obesity and its sequelae (for example, arthritis and diabetes) on the health of Americans.

Representing the aggregate disease burden of a population requires a measurement system that captures the effects of morbidity as well as mortality. Over the last 35 years, there has been substantial development of measures of health status and of health-related quality of life. Some of the measures are specific to particular organ systems. For example, the Arthritis Impact Measurement Scale considers the quality of life of people who have arthritis (Meenan et al., 1982). The 25-item National Eye Institute Vision Functioning Questionnaire records the effect of visual disturbance on functioning and quality of life (Mangione et al., 2001). Those disease-specific measures are well validated and used clinically, but they do not allow assessments of the relative contributions of particular diseases or conditions to the overall health of populations. For example, effects on functional limitation on the basis of pain and on the basis of visual deficit cannot be captured with the same measure. In addition, comorbidities increase as a population ages, and disease-specific measures cannot chart the cumulative impact of arthritis, visual impairment, and obesity.

To address those limitations, generic measures that are not tied to any disease or condition have been developed. Under the umbrella of HALYs are quality-adjusted life years (QALYs) and disability-adjusted life years

(DALYs), both of which allow the quantification of effects of disease and social determinants on health and permit the study of how clinical care and population-based interventions can alter them. Although both QALYs and DALYs create combined estimates of morbidity and mortality, the functions they were originally envisioned as serving—DALYs to capture global burden of disease, and QALYs as an outcome measure in cost-effectiveness studies—led to different approaches to capturing their morbidity aspects (Gold et al., 2002). From a practical perspective, both are currently used to serve either function, but in the United States and in Canada, the dominant form of HALY in use is the QALY.

QALYs are built from descriptive systems that include dimensions of function and symptomatology that are widely understood (e.g., in different cultural contexts) to characterize the varying effects of disease and disability on functioning. Health-related quality of life (HRQL) measures combine two sources of information: health states and health weights. Health states categorize levels of functioning in domains that include physical activity, mobility, pain, cognition, and mental state. Once a particular health state is described with respect to levels of function in different domains, information is collected from a representative sample of the community to weight the value of the health state relative to others. The point of the weighting is to capture the desirability of the health state (composed of many domains at levels of function) with a single number that can allow comparisons among diseases and conditions. Different techniques are used to aggregate responses into a single number on a 0–1 scale (where 0 = death and 1 = perfect health) that represents the average value of that health state in a population. The weight associated with a particular health state is the average of the preferences for that state in a sample of people in the community (Gold et al., 1996).

As with life expectancy, the average HRQL of different populations and across all health conditions can be examined on the basis of geography, demography, and other environmental and social determinants of health. The HRQL of a representative sample of Americans has been shown to be higher in groups that have more education and income and is inversely related to age (Lubetkin et al., 2005).

In the final step in creating summary measures of population health, the life expectancy of a population is combined with its HRQL to create "health-adjusted life expectancy" (HALE). (For a more detailed accounting, see Asada, 2010; Erickson, 1998; Gold and Muennig, 2002; Gold et al., 1996; IOM, 1998; Murray and Lopez, 2000; Murray et al., 2000; Pearcy and Keppel, 2002; Stiefel et al., 2010.) The relationships of the different indicators are illustrated in Figure 3-1.

HALE and HALYs represent the effects of any health condition and allow aggregation across all the conditions that can affect a population.

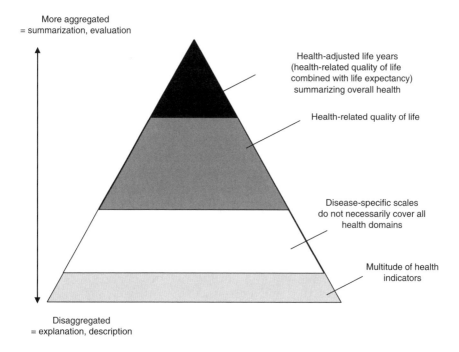

More aggregated
= summarization, evaluation

Health-adjusted life years
(health-related quality of life
combined with life expectancy)
summarizing overall health

Health-related quality of life

Disease-specific scales
do not necessarily cover all
health domains

Multitude of health
indicators

Disaggregated
= explanation, description

FIGURE 3-1 Data pyramid for population health.
SOURCE: Fryback, 2010, adapted from Wolfson.

They can provide information on the effects of particular illnesses, such as diabetes or cancer, on the health of a population (Boswell-Purdy et al., 2007; Manuel and Schultz, 2004). They can provide insight into regional differences associated with behavioral risk factors, such as smoking levels (Jia and Lubetkin, 2010). They can also allow examination of the health experiences of subpopulations by race and ethnicity and of exposure to different social and environmental risk factors. For example, using an HRQL measure from the Medical Expenditures Panel Survey and linked mortality data, Muennig and coauthors studied a number of social and behavioral risk factors and found that poverty, smoking, and high school dropout rates imposed the greatest burden of disease on Americans (Muennig et al., 2010). That study adds to the growing literature that has demonstrated the larger inequalities that race and socioeconomic status exact when measurement accounts for both health status and longevity (Franks et al., 2006; McIntosh et al., 2009; Muennig et al., 2005).

Over the last decade, use of the HALE and HALY summary measures has grown in both domestic and international clinical care and population health (e.g., policy) settings. Because of their ability to paint an overall pic-ture of the health of a community or a country, they have been referred to as a gross domestic product (GDP) for the health sector (see, for example, IOM, 1998; Wolfson, 1999).

Despite their versatility, HALYs and QALYs are not routinely used in health and health-system monitoring in the United States. Uptake has been slow in part because of the disparate approaches taken to measurement of the HRQL aspect of HALYs. However, recent work has shown relative concordance in outcomes of studies that compared existing measures, and a group of academics and policy-makers has called on the field to designate a measure that can be used in different types of population health and clini-cal care studies, as has been done in England and in Canada (Drummond et al., 2009). In addition, decision-makers have been leery of summary measures, largely because of the use of QALYs as an outcome measure for cost-effectiveness studies. In policy debates that date back to the Oregon Medicaid experiment (Kaplan, 1994), QALYs have been represented vari-ously as discriminating against people who are disadvantaged on the basis of disability, age, and social position because they stand to gain fewer HALYs from life-saving interventions than would accrue to people who are in better health or have longer life expectancy (Harris, 1987; Rawles, 1989). That view has been countered by others who have noted that cost-effectiveness analyses that use QALYs as outcome indicators do so from the perspective of a general population and do not evaluate economic efficiency on the basis of subpopulation characteristics (Russell et al., 1996). In the ACA, however, the new Patient-Centered Outcomes Institute is prohibited from using a "dollars per quality adjusted life year (or similar measure that discounts the value of a life because of an individual's disability) as a threshold to establish what type of health care is cost effective or recommended" (Garber and Sox, 2010; Neumann and Weinstein, 2010).

Although summary measures of population health like QALYs are prominent in discussions of rationing and the debate around the approach to curtailing clinical care costs, the uses of HALYs are far broader, permit-ting methods for monitoring health and for forecasting or directly studying the effects of different health and clinical interventions on communities and subpopulations. In public health settings, such as the Los Angeles County Health Department, DALYs have been used to provide information to sup-port priority-setting (Kominski et al., 2002, 2010). More recently, Wash-ington state has been using QALYs in priority-setting for population health (personal communication, A. Mokhdad, 2010).

In 1990, the HHS Healthy People initiative stated as its first goal "Im-prove Years of Healthy Life for all Americans"—a health-adjusted life ex-pectancy indicator (HHS et al., 2001). Lacking an agreed-on measure with which to track years of healthy life, NCHS created a composite placeholder measure with the intent of developing a more enduring approach for future use (Erickson et al., 1989; Gold et al., 2002).

Although this placeholder measure has not yet been replaced in national data sets, a growing understanding of the value of overall health measures has led to recent work by NCHS staff with international colleagues representing government and health organizations to identify and test concepts of health and function that are meaningful across countries and cultures (Taskforce on Health Status, 2005; The United Nations, 2010). The work of standing international committees (the Budapest Initiative and the Washington Group) has led to testing of measures that can be used to track progress and make comparisons internationally (see Box 3-1 for more details) (Madans, 2009; WHO et al., 2007). Questions on function—in domains that include vision, hearing, cognition, self-care, mobility, pain, fatigue, anxiety, and depression—are being tested on a sample from the 2010 NHIS, and the plan is to include a selected set on the full sample in 2011. The international working groups have identified the need to develop a "principled" weighting system derived from an empirical foundation or other agreed-on theory-based analytic technique that will unite the individual concepts of function into a summary measure. A measure arising from those efforts, which has been vetted by international and US measurement experts and is used at the national level, offers a model for building a

---

BOX 3-1
The Budapest Initiative and the Washington Group

The Budapest Initiative (originally called the Task Force on Measuring Health Status) held its first meeting in 2005 and is a collaborative effort involving national statistics offices and other international organizations working in health statistics with the objective of developing internationally comparable measures of health states. The measures could be used to develop a core set of health indicators for use at the local, national, and international levels (Taskforce on Health Status, 2005).

The purposes of the Washington Group (established in 2002) are to

- Foster international cooperation in health and disability statistics.
- Resolve the confusing and conflicting disability estimates internationally.
- Develop a small set of general disability measures.
- Develop extended sets of items to measure disability in population surveys.
- Address methodologic issues associated with disability measurement (Madans, 2008).

standardized measure of population health that can eventually be deployed at all levels of community.

In addition to functioning as outcome variables that permit building an evidence base for programs and policies, summary measures of population health hold potential for capturing public attention with respect to the health of their communities. The 1998 Institute of Medicine (IOM) report *Summarizing Population Health* (IOM, 1998) suggested that a broader understanding of the meaning of the measures would be helpful in alerting all Americans to the health experience of the United States and their own communities. Because the HALYs of a community represent the combined health experiences of its members (rather than a disease-by-disease characterization, as many current measures do), clear differentials among communities provide an overall picture of the health fortunes of a region or a subpopulation. Concerted efforts that familiarize Americans with the meaning of the measures, such as portraying them in terms of the "GDP of health," will be a key step in building the understanding that can galvanize action in and on behalf of populations and communities where health disparities are prominent.

The committee echoes the finding of prior work from IOM (IOM, 1998, 2003, 2006, 2009) and others that use of HALYs and life expectancy will markedly advance tools for tracking the health of populations and understanding what influences it. By embedding the building blocks with which to calculate HALE and HALYs in routine data-collection efforts at all geographic levels, the health system can gain a greater understanding of the effects of clinical care, population health interventions, and social policies on the health of the nation, its communities, and subpopulations that have been historically at higher risk for poorer health outcomes. As the most distal outcome measure (see Figure 3-2) in a coherent data system, HALE

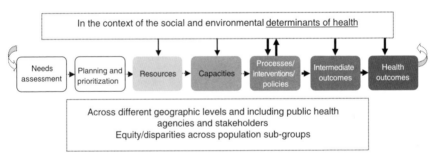

FIGURE 3-2 From inputs to outputs logic model.
NOTE: The thickness of some arrows denotes the present report's focus on those interactions.

and HALYs allow the building of models that can inform predictions and assessments of how investments in different parts of the health system will contribute to the health of the nation.

Public health professionals would use summary measures of population health to track changes in their communities and evaluate the success of particular initiatives over the long term inasmuch as population health changes slowly. One way that a summary measure was used in the past was as one of the top three goals of the Healthy People 2000 initiative—to "increase years of healthy life for all Americans"—a goal that was tracked throughout the initiative's implementation. Public health workers can also use summary measures, such as HALYs, to set priorities for resource expenditures by determining, for example, whether an obesity-related initiative that cost a given amount could improve HALYs by a particular percentage and would constitute a better investment than pursuing an injury-prevention (or other) program. Interventions that target different outcomes are not mutually exclusive, and the example provided is only an illustration of the type of use to which HALYs may be put. By conducting a "what if" analysis (for example, modeling with HALYs), a community might find that a particular type of investment in population-based initiatives could generate a particular number of HALYs at a particular cost and thus save money in the clinical care delivery system.

The committee finds that the nation's health statistics and information system lacks the categories of measures that could support the information needs of policy-makers, public health officials, health-system partners, and communities. No category of measure tells the complete story or offers a complete picture of health in the nation and in the community, and they each have limitations (for example, HALE needs to be disaggregated to allow understanding of reasons for disparities among localities, nations, and subpopulations and identification of more specific, actionable factors). But HALE and HALYs, community-health indicators, and outcome indicators complement each other as tools to inform and to galvanize action.

Recommendation 2
The committee recommends that the Department of Health and Human Services support and implement the following to integrate, align, and standardize health data and health-outcome measurement at all geographic levels:
a. A core, standardized set of indicators that can be used to assess the health of communities.

   b. A core, standardized set of health-outcome indicators for national, state, and local use.[6]
   c. A summary measure of population health that can be used to estimate and track health-adjusted life expectancy for the United States.

Ideally, these activities will be conducted with advice from a fully resourced and strengthened NCHS (see Recommendation 1) and will include systematic, periodic review of indicators to ensure their sustained relevance and usefulness.

The committee was not constituted to and did not endeavor to develop lists of proposed indicators. The process of developing and reaching evidence-based consensus on standardized indicator sets will require considerable research, broad-based dialogue (involving all relevant parties), and prioritization to come up with a parsimonious set. Research would include modeling and other efforts to elucidate the linked nature of many determinants of health and intermediate indicators of health where provision of information can lead to actionable measures at all geographic levels. A national effort to accomplish this may initially require defining a modest core set that all localities would be encouraged to use (e.g., to support comparisons and allow "rolling up" from the local to the state and even the national level), additional optimal indicators could be identified for other outcomes or community characteristics of interest to some localities.

The process of developing and reaching evidence-based consensus on indicator sets will require considerable research (including modeling and other efforts to clarify the complex, overlapping pathways between the many determinants of health and population health outcomes and the interrelated effects of interventions), dialogue, and prioritization to come up with reasonably sized sets of indicators. As has been often noted, one of the challenges of the Healthy People process has been the lengthy list of objectives and indicators, which may contribute to the difficulties of communicating, tracking, and reporting on progress in meeting them. HHS has been examining ways to streamline Healthy People and make it a more useful tool for planning (see, for example, NORC, 2005). (See Table 3-1 for sample outcome indicators and indicators of community health.)

---

[6] The conception of a community may differ from one context to another, and it could range from a neighborhood to a county. Local decision-makers may include mayors, boards of supervisors, and public health officials. The notion of local may also vary (from census tract or ZIP code to city or county) depending on planning or research objectives and many other factors.

TABLE 3-1 Sample (Distal) Outcome Indicators and Indicators of Community Health

Categories of Indicators	Examples
Community health (indicators of the health of the community itself—refers partly to indicators of determinants of health in local contexts)	Walkability Food insecurity Fresh-food availability Safety (gun-associated violence) Cohesion, social capital, social networks Inequity (e.g., data on distribution of clinical care, civic engagement, discrimination [real and perceived], education, and risk behaviors are accessible) Educational attainment, such as average years of schooling Physical environment (safe communities, diverse ecosystems, climate change, toxic exposures, health-promoting exposures)
Health outcomes (mostly distal, but also behavioral risk factors; aggregate indicators of individual health or health risk and risky behavior)	Smoking rates Cardiovascular disease Disease-specific mortality Infant mortality Life expectancy Asthma Health or functional status Health-adjusted life expectancy

ADOPTING THE DETERMINANTS OF HEALTH PERSPECTIVE AT A FUNDAMENTAL LEVEL

The inputs-to-outputs logic model provided in Chapter 2 (see Figure 3-2), showing how steps in the population health improvement process are connected, illustrates the feedback loop between processes or interventions that modify determinants of health, which in turn become improved intermediate outcomes. The logic model also highlights the importance of understanding the causal relationships and interrelationships among the health outcomes, determinants, and evidence-based interventions.

Individual characteristics (e.g., genetics, sociodemographics, and health behaviors), community characteristics (physical and social environment), and clinical care all contribute to the total health of a community, a state, or a nation. The aggregated experience of individual people in health-related quality of life and longevity was viewed by the committee as the common distal health outcome that the health system works to maximize.

Chapter 2 described the categories on the far right of the logic model as having more indicators available (for example, on disease-specific outcomes, data such as rates of cardiovascular disease [CVD] and cancer incidence) than those on the left. Also, some of the data that exist on the left side of the continuum (on capacities, performance) is found in the clinical care context—illustrating yet another reason for sharing and collaborating between the clinical care and public health communities. Those on the right side, however, typically draw on data from sources oriented toward the medical model and generally lack a determinants-of-health orientation in their reporting. Many categories of determinants of health are not measured by government-sponsored population health surveys, as this report has discussed in the section on the need for community health indicators. Information that is central to understanding health and promoting action to improve it often resides in government databases outside HHS or in the private sector. Examples of the former include information maintained by agencies in the US Department of Agriculture (the sources used in the department's *Food Environment Atlas*), the Department of Commerce (Bureau of the Census data sets, such as the American Housing Survey and the American Community Survey), the Department of Transportation (the National Household Transportation Survey), the Bureau of Economic Analysis, and the Bureau of Labor Statistics (the Current Population Survey). Examples of the latter include data available from the food industry, retailers, local authorities, Web search engines, and other consumer- and industry-focused services (see, for example, Brownson et al., 2005). Making explicit the different contributions of many sectors to the social and environmental determinants of health demonstrates the need for sharing, linking, and integrating data that suggest opportunities and provide a more complete picture of the health of a community. That will require a broadening of the array of information available through public–public and public–private collaborations.

The committee believes that a national conversation is needed to transform how Americans conceptualize the factors that influence health outcomes and to demonstrate the potential contributions of moving beyond the medical model toward an ecologic, population-based approach to health improvement. It would afford clinical care the weight it merits as well as heighten understanding of the myriad other loci available for action. Other wealthy nations brief their populations on the social and environmental determinants of health, and such efforts are intended to heighten awareness and promote action that leads to improved health and health equity. International efforts that examine health status include the Human Development reports of the World Bank and the work of the World Health Organization.

National dialogue about health in such nations as Canada and the United Kingdom (UK) routinely includes references to determinants of health and to inequalities in health status that are related to socioeconomic status (for an overview of these issues, see Chapter 1). For example, the Canadian

Senate's Subcommittee on Population Health released a report (2009) titled *A Healthy, Productive Canada: A Determinant of Health Approach*. The report listed the multiple determinants of the health of Canadians (housing, physical environment, early childhood environment, education, income and social status, employment and working conditions, and culture and sex) and showed that clinical care—on which Canada, like the United States, out-spends many peer nations—alone cannot improve health outcomes. Other, older contributions to the higher profile of social and economic factors outside the United States include the UK's Acheson report on inequalities in health and their causes (Lowdell et al., 1999) and the Canadian report by Evans and colleagues titled *Why Are Some People Healthy and Others Not? The Determinants of Health of Populations* (1990). Another relevant report was prepared by the Commission on the Measurement of Economic Performance and Social Progress at the request of French President Nicolas Sarkozy. In that report, Stiglitz and colleagues (2009) responded to the concern that France was overrelying on the GDP as an indicator of national well-being. Stiglitz et al. showed the need for and importance of other in-dicators both to inform the nation on its progress and to spur change, and they proposed new approaches, such as transforming statistical systems, to measure the dimensions of well-being, including health, and to comple-ment what the GDP shows about a nation's trajectory. The British report *Fair Society, Healthy Lives: A Strategic Review of Health Inequalities in England Post* (The Marmot Review, 2010) provides another example of a major government-commissioned report that is being rolled out throughout the UK and is intended to lead to "developing policies, building capacity and recommending practical steps to address the social determinants of health."

A high-visibility annual report that describes the health of Americans on the basis of sociodemographics and other social and environmental determinants is a missing element in changing this nation's narrative on health. As we gain further understanding of community-level indicators that directly influence the health of individuals, increasingly rich information on social and environmental determinants of health can be made available at national, state, and local levels. Wide dissemination of this sort would allow people everywhere to better understand the forces that create and detract from health in communities and thereby drive responses and actions appro-priate to local conditions. Compilation of such data is resource-intensive, however, and some of the information is not available in many localities. An immediate and feasible first step would be to produce a national report that regularly updates and highlights the nation's health, focusing on a determinants model.

Recommendation 3
The committee recommends that the Department of Health and
Human Services produce an annual report to inform policy-makers,
all health-system sectors, and the public about important trends
and disparities in social and environmental determinants that
affect health.

A strengthened and adequately resourced NCHS could play a central
role in the development of such a report. The report would require some
additional infrastructure to accomplish the secondary research, analyses,
and other activities. In addition, although the report would presumably
include state-level data, large metropolitan areas would ideally be included.
Undertaking such an effort would require financial and human resources,
but the committee was unable to examine these in any detail.

RESPONSIVENESS TO THE NEEDS OF END USERS

Some aspects of responsiveness to the need of decision-makers and
communities would be addressed by implementation of Recommendations
1 and 2, pertaining to strengthening NCHS to play a greater leadership role
in the nation's population health information and statistics system, and to
the development and implementation of a summary measure of population health and two standardized sets of indicators. Below, the committee
provides rationale for and offers two recommendations that pertain both to
the population health-clinical care interface and to the overarching need for
modeling and related research to support information needs. The discussion
of modeling also points back to the earlier discussion about the determinants
of health; the field's understanding of how these influence health could be
greatly enhanced through modeling and related analyses.

One of the challenges facing the population health information system
is intersectoral information exchange, coordination, and collaboration,
including the interface between public health agencies and the clinical care
delivery system but extending to education, transportation, and other fields
in which public-sector and private-sector decisions can affect population
health.

The interface between the clinical care system and public health agencies is a major potential source of valuable information on population
health, but, as discussed below, various concerns must first be addressed.
Some information pertinent to population health and not available from
national population health data sets may be obtained from clinical care
sources, including information on chronic-disease prevalence and prevention, prevalence of a wide array of diseases, and functional status (HHS et
al., 2002; Luck et al., 2006; NCVHS, 2010). Public health agencies interact

with the clinical care system in various ways, in addition to providing some primary-care services themselves. The interactions may take the form of surveillance for reportable diseases, vital records, and statutorily established regulatory roles for selected state public health agencies, such as licensing and certification of hospitals and nursing homes. Some state and local public health agencies also perform the role of health-information stewards, analysts, and technical advisers, collecting population health–relevant data from providers in a community and conducting supporting activities to help providers to improve their performance and patient outcomes. It should be noted that some public health agencies are combined with or include departments that oversee clinical services, whereas others are separate from departments charged with clinical care assurance. One example of a clinically oriented public health program may be found in New York City, where the Department of Health and Mental Hygiene has established a hemoglobin A1C registry that mandates laboratory reporting of hemoglobin A1C test results, involves over 1,000 providers, and is designed to improve diabetes management in the city (Chamany et al., 2009). As another example, New York State has had a coronary-artery-bypass-surgery registry in place since 1989. Its intent is twofold: to provide information to clinical care teams and hospitals for quality improvement, and to alert the public about which centers are the best performers (Hannon and Beach, 1994). At the national level, the Centers for Medicare and Medicaid Services (CMS) began tracking "never" events (medical errors and untoward outcomes that should never occur, such as wrong-site surgery, bedsores, and hospital-associated infections) and began denying payment for any clinical services provided to address such events.

Immunization registries are an early form of a population health information system designed for a specific purpose and overseen by public health agencies of states and large cities. Immunization-information systems receive data from and provide data to the full array of immunization providers, including private clinical practices, federally qualified health centers, and public health clinics. In areas where health-information exchanges are operational—such as Indiana, Michigan, and Rhode Island—public health agencies become involved in the exchange. Regional health-information organizations have been organized in several areas to rationalize and facilitate secure health-information exchange among providers in a community or region, including public health agency clinic health-information systems.

In building a coherent data system that monitors health and evaluates interventions and policies that improve it, the clinical care system has much to contribute to the health-information system. Reporting of particular types of data from the clinical care delivery system to public health can accomplish two major functions:

- Conducting population-based surveillance and assessment by providing information that can be uniquely and efficiently gathered
  in the clinical care system to form a more complete picture of the
  health of a community and the people in it.
- Monitoring the quality and safety of clinical care services to provide
  information that can enhance performance and accountability of
  the clinical care system (this includes enhancing the use of clinical
  preventive services to address such risk factors as smoking and
  effective management of chronic diseases with the greatest population impact and preventing harm that can arise in the clinical care
  setting).

Population-Based Surveillance and the Clinical Care System

Population-based surveillance and information can be transmitted
bidirectionally between the public health and clinical care delivery systems
to help each fulfill its mission and target its activities better. For example,
although it is financially daunting to mount a health-examination survey
in every community, some key information already present in the clinical
care system in many communities can be used to assess the prevalence and
control of diabetes, hypertension, and hyperlipidemia and the use of clinical
preventive services. The current state of data-sharing between public health
agencies and medical care organizations varies greatly from one jurisdiction
to another, and data-sharing is poorly standardized. For example, most
state public health agencies use an immunization-information system (or
registry), but participation of clinical care providers in the system may range
from 100 percent to far smaller proportions, especially in communities that
have many independent practices with little access to technology. Some 75
percent of public and 37 percent of private immunization providers partici-
pate in registries (Hinman and Ross, 2010). In addition to immunization
registries, cancer registries and disease- and injury-reporting systems (such
as the National Electronic Injury Surveillance System: Cooperative Adverse
Drug Events Surveillance System) provide examples of the public health
use of clinical data. Those systems serve important public health purposes,
but they also present challenges. For example, because of the nature of
their structure (organized in vertical programmatic "silos" without optimal
coordination), they place additional reporting burdens on the clinical care
system, requiring partially redundant data collection and reporting or requiring entry of different types of diagnoses into multiple databases rather
than into an integrated, multipurpose database.

The increased emphasis on and support of electronically collected and
stored information in the clinical care delivery system creates rich opportunities. For example, data obtainable from electronic health records (EHRs)

include claims for services and medications and laboratory data and could be integrated with or superimposed on information from population surveys that estimate prevalence on the basis of such questions as, "Has a doctor or a nurse ever told you that you have diabetes?"

The committee was mindful that use of electronic information creates procedural and logistical challenges. One logistical challenge arises because many people see a variety of providers who may not be electronically linked. Several other challenges arise from the ability of public health agencies to access medical care data for public health purposes. However, those data may not be accessible at the interface between providers and their patients, and there may be serious concerns related to privacy, right of access, and intended use of personal data. A different type of problem emerges from reporting of notifiable diseases. Such reporting has become markedly streamlined with direct reporting of results by laboratories and emergency rooms to the public health infrastructure. However, public health agencies and all partners in the health system must maintain caution to avoid the pitfalls of this more complete access, including the potential of spending more time and energy in collecting data than in using it thoughtfully.

Clinical care data can contribute substantially to public health agencies' knowledge of population health and enhance their ability to identify and solve community health problems. This is also Essential Public Health Service #1—"monitor health status to identify and solve community health problems"—as described in Ten Essential Public Health Services developed by the Core Public Health Functions Steering Committee in 1994. Also, public health agencies can provide denominator data that can be helpful to clinicians. However, barriers exist to data-sharing and collaboration, and solutions must be identified. Although there are great hopes for the universal implementation of EHRs, their existence alone does not remove the obstacles to making needed population-based information widely available.[7] Both thought and resources need to be put into defining what information is best harvested from the clinical system and how it should be obtained. Simply providing open-ended clinical care data to public health authorities will not be acceptable to the clinical care system or the public. Other considerations and barriers to unrestricted use and sharing of this information with the broader health system in a community include the following:

---

[7] One interesting example to improve quality of care through use of EHRs is the Primary Care Information Project (PCIP) in New York City, which "seeks to improve the quality of care in underserved communities through the use of health information technology," including the adoption of quality EHRs and an "agenda of prevention" (New York City Department of Health and Mental Hygiene, 2009).

- Health departments are, in general, authorized to receive confidential information from clinical sources for public health purposes. They are also generally required to keep such information confidential, so information released to other parties must be stripped of any potentially identifying information.
- Public health surveillance is regarded as "practice," not "research," and so is not subject to consideration by institutional review boards or informed-consent requirements, although public health agencies recognize the importance of appropriate use and safeguards of the data to protect privacy and confidentiality. Analyses conducted by nongovernment entities are subject to different constraints.
- Information that can be linked back to providers, clinical care systems, or insurance companies may be viewed as proprietary by those providers or systems and therefore less likely to be reported if released publicly in a way that maintains that link. Related concerns stem from the potential effects of data-sharing on reimbursement and medicolegal liability.
- Key information useful for understanding population health—such as race, ethnicity, and educational achievement—might not be routinely collected by providers, and its collection might entail extra cost and effort. However, the Health Information Technology for Economic and Clinical Health Act requires the collection of demographic information for payment.

Great care will be needed to change the current state with legislation, funding, logistics, and technology and to define the attributes of the mechanisms for maximizing the use and usefulness of clinical care data to health-system stakeholders.

For data-sharing to be successful, it is critical that benefit flow from government public health agencies to clinical care stakeholders. For example, providers of clinical care need easier access to their own data that are submitted to government entities (federal, state, or local), access to analyses to help them benchmark and improve the appropriateness of the care they deliver, and access to other population health data (such as disparities and determinants) that are pertinent to the groups they serve so they can tailor their clinical care and community services to the population served to meet needs and improve outcomes.

The committee agrees with others who have commented on the actual and potential value of clinical care system data to inform population health efforts, including filling gaps in data available from other sources (NCVHS, 2010). The Office of the National Coordinator for Health Information Technology has emphasized the importance of including public health and population health goals in its various activities, and continued attention from relevant groups will be needed to assure that investments in e-health initiatives do consider the population health and public health relevance of electronic health records and related efforts.

Recommendation 4
The committee recommends that governmental public health agencies partner with medical care organizations and providers in their jurisdictions to share information[8] derived from clinical-data sources, when appropriate, to inform relevant population health priorities. Such information will support core health indicators that are otherwise unavailable at some or all geographic levels.

Indicators shared in that way may include prevalence data on traditional risk factors (such as smoking, lack of physical activity, and hypertension) and measures of preventive-service delivery and chronic-disease control. Other indicators that help in assessing the readiness of the community to interact with the clinical care delivery system in an informed manner might be added to the clinical data collected. They include measures of health literacy (Adams, 2010; DeWalt et al., 2004) and patient activation (Hibbard et al., 2004; Mancuso and Rincon, 2006; Paasche-Orlow and Wolf, 2007). Both health literacy and patient activation are known to influence outcomes in the clinical setting favorably (Adams, 2010; Hibbard et al., 2004).

The use of EHRs has accelerated in recent years, owing in part to such federal government initiatives as the creation of the Office of the National Coordinator of Health Information Technology in HHS and funding through the American Recovery and Reinvestment Act. At the state level, Minnesota has set deadlines for universal adoption of EHRs by all hospitals and clinical care providers (Mayberry and Hunkins, 2008). EHRs raise questions about equity, generalizability, and overreporting, and the use of clinical care data for population health purposes presents considerable concerns related to privacy and confidentiality (Safran, 2007). Although ample statutory protections are in place both for patients and for the public good, these related but discrete objectives (i.e., individual and societal needs) must be constantly held in balance, and all necessary actions to preserve this balance (and the credibility of all system components entrusted with personal identifying data) must be sustained with transparency and deliberation.

Clinical care data by definition include only information that is obtained in the clinical care system and are therefore not equivalent to population-based data. Although EHRs are limited in their ability to capture undetected

---

[8] Information shared will generally be deidentified and aggregated. In some circumstances, however, the data are and must be tracked individually (for example, for infectious-disease reporting and immunization-registry purposes). Variations in local needs and public health authority may lead to other types of data-use agreements.

disease in the community, they can provide some insights into the descriptive epidemiology of disease (Califf and Ginsburg, 2008). A later report on law by the present committee will explore this more fully; any public health role in monitoring clinical care quality and outcomes through the use of personal health information requires a broader discussion about the role of government and the scope of government involvement.

Monitoring Outcomes of the Clinical Care System

Monitoring of the outcomes of the clinical care system by public health agencies can provide critical information about appropriate use, overuse, underuse, and misuse of medical technologies and can make the clinical care delivery system more efficient. However, different jurisdictions might make different decisions regarding whether this function is best housed in government public health agencies.

The American clinical care system has extraordinary capabilities, but it is also inefficient and is itself the cause of adverse events (IOM, 2000; Orszag, 2008). Policy-makers and clinical care system leaders in both the public and the private sector are increasingly recognizing and seeking to address those serious challenges. The American public is generally unfamiliar with the related notions of evidence-based medicine and comparative effectiveness (and the clinical field's broader emphasis on improving quality, effectiveness, and efficiency). It is a sad testament both to the generally low levels of health literacy of the American public and to the unsuccessful efforts by the educational and clinical care systems and others to inform and educate the public (Clancy and Cronin, 2005; IOM, 2004). Many American patients assume that more clinical care is better care—for example, that care by specialists is generically better than that by primary-care providers, that more intensive treatments are more effective, or that the newest medical product is the best (Carman et al., 2010).

A variety of sources provide information on the quality and outcomes of clinical care in the United States. They include the Dartmouth Atlas Project, which "examines regional variations in the practice of medicine and in spending for health care, principally in the Medicare population" (Fisher et al., 2009); the *National Healthcare Quality Report* produced annually by the Agency for Healthcare Research and Quality; data sets and reports prepared by such clinical quality organizations as the National Committee for Quality Assurance, the National Quality Forum, and the Joint Commission; and a variety of reports produced by health plans and other medical-care organizations. However, much more (especially on the use of preventive care and on clinical care–associated harm) could be communicated to the public in an easy-to-understand format and in the context of a broader effort to inform and educate the public about effectiveness and efficiency in clinical

care and to support more informed decision-making by patients. The committee believes that public health agencies can play an important role in
reporting to the public on local clinical care system performance.

Research on the effects of public reporting of clinical care system performance, including quality of care, shows that its effects on consumers are
mixed. They depend on characteristics of consumers themselves, consumer
awareness of the availability of such information, the presentation and
clarity of the information, and its relevance to consumers' own information
needs, which are largely for information that is pertinent to their clinical
needs and to their providers and information about errors and adverse events
(Faber et al., 2009; Hibbard et al., 2005; Mosen et al., 2007; Schauffler and
Mordavsky, 2001). Although consumers are not always well informed, often
because available information is inaccessible to them, improving the clarity
and completeness of public information about the performance of the clinical care system with respect to issues of appropriateness of care (underuse,
overuse, and misuse), its quality, and its cost—with concerted efforts at
public education—can inform consumer decision-making and enhance understanding of the strengths and limitations of clinical care. Most current
indicators in the quality-improvement literature are "positive" indicators
(for example, for interventions that are underused rather than overused
or misused). That is understandable inasmuch as stakeholders can reach
consensus on what needs to be done more easily than on what is currently
done that should not be done.

Recommendation 5
The committee recommends that state and local public health agencies in each state collaborate with clinical care delivery systems to
assure that the public has greater awareness of the appropriateness,
quality, safety, and efficiency of clinical care services delivered in
their state and community. Local performance reports about overuse, underuse, and misuse should be made available for selected
interventions (including preventive and diagnostic tests, procedures,
and treatment).

Such collaboration is needed to support continuous quality improvement among clinical care providers and alert the community to the effectiveness of the medical-care delivery system. Also, the collaborative convening
of public health agencies and clinical care entities would likely include
activities such as the joint development of evidence-based indicators and
the development of a process to use data for system improvements, and
will require a strong assurance of the privacy and confidentiality of clinical
data to facilitate openness and collaboration. In settings where the public
health agency is the quality assurer or regulator, establishing collaborative

relationships with the clinical care delivery system may be more challenging or complex.

Systems-Based Modeling and Simulation

There is still much to be understood about causal pathways in health and about which indicators are most useful for fostering understanding of health and for informing and mobilizing action to improve it. Systems-based modeling and simulation, although characterized by some limitations, are important tools that can advance this work.

Models are simplified representations of real-world systems—including biologic, environmental, behavioral, and organizational factors—that help us to understand these systems and answer questions about them. Models not only provide a way to understand what happened in the past but also provide an ability to explore what might happen under conditions that have not occurred, such as how a hypothetical system might behave, or to assess the benefits and harms of policy options. Models advance measurement in several ways. First, the process of building a model highlights in an explicit and systematic manner the relationships of model components and the data needed to implement the model. That can ensure that the major components are included in the model and can identify data elements that are needed. When those data are unavailable, the process points to the need to collect additional data elements or forces a model to be reconceptualized. Second, after a simulation model is run, a variety of what-if scenarios, formal sensitivity analysis[9] (Fu, 2006), and factor-screening[10] (Shen and Wan, 2009) can be used to identify the most critical factors that affect the model outputs and hence the most important data needed to focus on these factors. Modeling and simulation have long been used in many fields to maximize performance, productivity, and effectiveness, allowing system designers, planners, and managers to test a broad array of what-if scenarios and situations—for example, in flight simulators, weather forecasting, manufacturing and services systems, and computer-aided design (Law, 2007; Mass et al., 2002).

Statistical and simulation models are increasingly used in clinical care and in the study of population health. Statistical models relate such input variables as age, exercise level, and caloric intake to such output variables as glycated hemoglobin, body mass index (BMI), and adverse events (Navarro-Barrientos et al., 2010). Public health agencies and investigators have used

---

[9] Formal sensitivity analysis uses key quantitative assumptions and computations (underlying a decision or estimate) that are changed systematically to assess their effect on the final outcome. "Employed commonly in evaluation of the overall risk or in identification of critical factors, it attempts to predict alternative outcomes of the same course of action" (Fu, 2006).

[10] "Factor screening is performed to eliminate unimportant factors so that the remaining important factors can be more thoroughly studied in later experiments" (Shen and Wan, 2009).

modeling for numerous objectives, including prediction of the spread and control of infectious diseases and examination of the relationship of such behaviors and health outcomes as alcohol use and motor-vehicle injuries and such environmental exposures as air pollution and associated morbidity in people who have pulmonary diseases (Epstein, 2009; Kim and Neff, 2010; Peng et al., 2008; Pope et al., 2009). Modeling may serve as a tool for examining what-if scenarios when empirical outcome data are lacking or not generalizable. For example, if evidence of the effectiveness of an intervention in reducing obesity is lacking, the business community, health plans, or CMS may still wish to determine how much of a BMI reduction needs to be achieved by any intervention to produce a return on a hypothetical investment in 5 years under a given set of assumptions. A model could inform decision-makers that they will need the public health community to develop an intervention that might, for example, produce a 4 percent or greater reduction in BMI to offset their costs. Researchers could then be tasked with developing and testing strategies to reach that goal.

Modeling allows decision-makers to consider many aspects of the complex and interconnected causal pathways that lead to poor health outcomes, such as infant mortality or heart disease. As shown by the "problem tree"–style illustrations in Chapter 2 that highlight the difference between a largely clinical approach and a population and ecologic root-causes approach to CVD and infant mortality, intermediate outcomes (blood pressure decreases, smoking cessation, and amelioration or removal of other risk factors) and stakeholder actions that are intended to improve one outcome often have effects on multiple health outcomes. For example, increasing high school graduation rates is associated both with improvements in distal health outcomes (such as decreased infant mortality and decreased CVD) and with improvements in risk profiles (for example, decreased smoking rates and increased physical activity) that influence health-related quality of life, life expectancy, and, ultimately, HALYs. Models can consider health behaviors, social characteristics, and systems variables and suggest what can happen if variables change. As the evidence base grows, new variables and indicators can be introduced into models to continue to build understanding.

Statistical models can be useful for predictive purposes, but generally the underlying assumption of such models is that past trends and relationships can predict future behavior. That assumption may not be appropriate in trying to predict effects for a system like health, which receives inputs from an increasing array of sources and which evolves over time (Pearl, 2000). System-dynamics models have therefore been applied in health; they permit diverse variables in multiple sectors to change dynamically and to change each other. They have been used effectively in population health to optimize vaccination policies for HIV (Brandeau and Zaric, 2009) and for hepatitis B viruses (Hutton et al., 2007), to understand the effects of differ-

BOX 3-2
Health Impact Assessments (HIAs)

A current IOM committee, the Committee on Health Impact Assessment, is developing a report that will explain the rationale of HIAs, enumerate their core elements and activities in the HIA process, describe the current practice, and provide guidance and provoke further exploration on effective HIA practice (expected to be released in 2011[a]). An overview of HIAs and a few examples are provided below.

An HIA is commonly defined as "a combination of procedures, methods, and tools by which a policy, program, or project may be judged as to its potential effects on the health of a population, and the distribution of those effects within the population" (WHO and ECHP, 1999).

An HIA is implemented before a project or policy is put into action to determine its potential health effects objectively. It brings together information from sectors beyond public health (such as transportation) to help in the decision-making process. It focuses on health outcomes, such as obesity, physical inactivity, asthma, injuries, and social equity (CDC, 2010b).

The major steps in conducting an HIA include (CDC, 2010b):

- Screening (identify projects or policies for which an HIA would be useful).
- Scoping (identify which health effects to consider).
- Assessing risks and benefits (identify which people may be affected and how they may be affected).
- Developing recommendations (suggest changes to proposals to promote favorable or mitigate adverse health effects).
- Reporting (present the results to decision-makers).
- Evaluating (determine the effect of the HIA on the decision).

ent interventions on pandemic outbreaks (Epstein, 2009; Ford et al., 2006), to study consumer eating behavior (Hammond, 2008), for cancer-screening optimization (Subramanian et al., 2010), and even for public health planning (Homer et al., 2007). Health impact assessments (HIAs) use a variety of modeling techniques to assess the benefits and harms of policy options—for example, the effects of living-wage laws, land use, and menu labeling (UCLA HIA-CLIC, 2010) (see Box 3-2 for more information on HIAs). Examining and leveraging existing simulation models would be useful. For example, the National Collaborative on Childhood Obesity Research has partnered with CDC, the National Institutes of Health (NIH), the Robert Wood Johnson Foundation, and the US Department of Agriculture to "forecast the impact of public health policies and interventions on childhood obesity on a population-wide level and among specific subpopulations" to simulate health

There are many ways in which an HIA can be implemented; depending on the method and tools used, they can be completed in a few days or take several months (Cole et al., 2005). HIA is used in Canada, Europe, Australia, and New Zealand; for some it is part of the regulatory process, for others it is voluntary (CDC, 2010b; Cole and Fielding, 2007; Cole et al., 2005). Several state legislatures—including those of California, Maryland, and Massachusetts—are considering bills that would implement HIA. The following are examples of HIA use in the United States:

- The San Francisco Department of Public Health regularly uses HIA to analyze community issues and provides education and training on HIA (City and County of San Francisco Department of Public Health, 2010).
- The White House Task Force on Childhood Obesity recommended that communities consider using HIA as part of their decision-making process (White House Task Force on Childhood Obesity, 2010).
- In Hawaii, the Department of Agriculture is partnering with Kaiser Permanente, the Center for Health Research, Human Impact Partners, and the Kohala Center to develop an HIA that will inform the development of a County of Hawaii Agriculture Development Plan, which is in response to the loss of sugar plantations that once dominated the economy (The Kohala Center, 2008).

For more information, see CDC Healthy Places (CDC, 2010a), Dannenberg et al. (2006), Health Impact Assessment Gateway (APHO, 2007), and the WHO Health Impact Assessment (WHO, 2010).

---

[a] See http:www8.nationalacademies.org/cp/CommitteeView.aspx?key=49158 (accessed September 8, 2010).

outcomes and potential cost savings from alternative health-promotion interventions (NCCOR, 2010).

In Canada, government health statisticians have been using simulation modeling to project the health-status trajectories of a longitudinal sample of people to inform health priorities and policy decisions (Wolfson, 1999) (see Box 3-3 for an example of some single outcome-specific uses of modeling). Various risk-behavior states in the population are interrelated to multiple outcomes—for example, smoking and multiple types of cancers and cardiovascular diseases. In the United States, the NIH Office of Behavioral and Social Sciences Research is leading efforts to accelerate the use of systems-based modeling in health (Mabry et al., 2010). CDC has also embraced systems-based modeling to advance community-based intervention strategies. This form of analysis can identify common causes of coexisting and synergistic conditions, such as substance abuse, violence, and sexually

BOX 3-3
Examples of the Use of Modeling by Statistics Canada

The Population Health Model (POHEM) is a microsimulation model of diseases and risk factors in which the basic unit of analysis is the individual person. The simulation creates and ages a large sample population representative of Canada, one individual at a time, until death. The life trajectory of each simulated person unfolds by exposure to different life-like events, such as smoking initiation and cessation, changes in weight, and incidence and progression of such diseases as osteoarthritis, cancer, diabetes, and heart disease.

POHEM combines data from a wide array of sources, including nationally representative cross-sectional and longitudinal surveys, cancer registries, hospitalization databases, vital statistics, census, and treatment-cost data. The model inputs may be altered at the user's request to investigate what-if scenarios. The scenarios can be useful for policy-makers by providing information beyond what is available from retrospective population studies.

Earlier versions of POHEM were used to estimate lifetime costs of breast and colorectal cancer and for assessments of health technology in cancer control, such as chemotherapy options for advanced lung cancer, the use of preventive tamoxifen in Canadian women, and the impact of population-based colorectal-cancer screening.

More recent generations of POHEM models have been developed for other common diseases—such as osteoarthritis, acute myocardial infarction, and diabetes—and for disease risk factors, such as obesity and physical inactivity. The risk-factor modules enable users to simulate the effects of changes in obesity or physical activity on key health outcomes.[a]

---

[a] The examples above illustrate the more traditional applications of population health modeling, but more recent Canadian work has moved in the direction of exploring multiple variables (from behavioral risk factors to the broad determinants of health) and their effects on health outcomes, including health-adjusted life expectancy (Wolfson and Rowe, 2009). Michael Wolfson has highlighted the potential uses of a summary measure of population health but notes that the health-adjusted life expectancy of a population is a reflection of myriad factors, some of which can be influenced by public policy. Modeling can use data to explore the relationship of health-related policy to broad health outcomes. However, arriving at a more robust and evolving understanding of how to maximize the health of populations and subpopulations requires exploration of the effects of social, environmental, and other determinants.
SOURCE: Statistics Canada, 2010.

transmitted diseases (Milstein, 2008), that contribute to disease burdens in communities.

The complex, changing nature of the conditions (e.g., social, economic, environmental) that influence health, productivity, and the volume of patients flowing into the clinical care system requires increased use of analytic approaches that elucidate interactions and interdependences among different systems and sectors, such as those between the traditional health sector (clinical care and government public health) and transportation, employment, and education (Collins et al., 2009). The success of the United States in dramatically reducing mortality from motor-vehicle collisions is a good illustration of the effects on health of actions taken in other sectors. Despite the meteoric rises in the numbers of motor vehicles and of miles driven per person, motor-vehicle fatality rates declined precipitously throughout the second half of the 20th century. That was a result of system-wide and mutually reinforcing interventions ranging from vehicle-safety design to traffic management, road construction design, alcohol regulation and enforcement, seat-belt laws and enforcement, workplace substance-abuse policies, and numerous community-based programs, including designated-driver and family-oriented engagement initiatives (Bolen et al., 1997). The transformation of the Department of Veterans Affairs health care system in the 1990s provides an example of dramatic system-wide improvement occurring in a short time through use of overlapping and reinforcing change strategies, including integrating and coordinating services and creation of an accountable management structure (Kizer and Dudley, 2009). "Bending the curve" of effects of chronic diseases and injury on functioning, productivity, clinical care use, and cost will require better information to support systemic improvements. Insights from modeling are essential for improved decision-making regarding priorities for intervention, collaboration among health-system sectors, and resource allocations. However, modeling itself will require further development and research.

Recommendation 6
The committee recommends that the Department of Health and Human Services (HHS) coordinate the development and evaluation and advance the use of predictive and system-based simulation models to understand the health consequences of underlying determinants of health. HHS should also use modeling to assess intended and unintended outcomes associated with policy, funding, investment, and resource options.

CONCLUDING OBSERVATIONS

The need for better and consistent measures at all levels to inform those who work to improve the health of the nation is great. This chapter makes recommendations that, if implemented, will lead to a more coherent population health information and statistics system. Advancing the timeliness and usefulness of data by creating standards, addressing inefficiencies, aligning health objectives, and improving coordination is key to meeting that goal. Communication of data to policy-makers and the public can help to create a system in which decisions are made based on current information about the true health needs of the country, and actions are taken to confront health issues that will have the greatest impact.

REFERENCES

Adams, R. J. 2010. Improving health outcomes with better patient understanding and education. *Risk Management and Healthcare Policy* 3:61-72.

APHO (Association of Public Health Observatories). 2007. *The HIA Gateway.* http://www.hiagateway.org.uk (September 8, 2010).

Asada, Y. 2010. A summary measure of health inequalities for a pay-for-population health performance system. *Preventing Chronic Disease Public Health Research, Practice and Policy* 7(4). http://www.cdc.gov/pcd/issues/2010/jul/09_0250.htm (July 4, 2010).

Bolen, J. R., D. A. Sleet, and T. Chorba. 1997. Overview of efforts to prevent motor vehicle-related injury. In *Prevention of motor vehicle-related injuries: A compendium of articles from the morbidity and mortality weekly report, 1985-1996.* Washington, DC: HHS and CDC.

Boswell-Purdy, J., W. M. Flanagan, H. Roberge, C. Le Petit, K. J. White, and J. M. Berthelot. 2007. Population health impact of cancer in Canada, 2001. *Chronic Diseases in Canada* 28(1-2):42-55.

Brandeau, M., and G. Zaric. 2009. Optimal investment in HIV prevention programs: More is not always better. *Health Care Management Science* 12(1):27-37.

Brownson, R. C., T. K. Boehmer, and D. A. Luke. 2005. Declining rates of physical activity in the United States: What are the contributors? *Annual Review of Public Health* 26:421-443.

Califf, R. M., and G. S. Ginsburg. 2008. Organizational improvements to enhance modern clinical epidemiology. *Journal of the American Medical Association* 300(19):2300-2302.

Canadian Senate Subcommittee on Population Health. 2009. *A healthy, productive Canada: A determinant of health approach.* Ottawa, Canada.

Carman, K. L., M. Maurer, J. M. Yegian, P. Dardess, J. McGee, M. Evers, and K. O. Marlo. 2010. Evidence that consumers are skeptical about evidence-based health care. *Health Affairs* 29(7):1400-1406.

CDC (Centers for Disease Control and Prevention). 2009. *The NCHS Mission.* http://www.cdc.gov/nchs/about/mission.htm (November 3, 2010).

CDC. 2010a. *Designing and Building Healthy Places.* http://www.cdc.gov/healthyplaces/ (September 8, 2010).

CDC. 2010b. *Healthy Places: Health Impact Assessment.* http://www.cdc.gov/healthyplaces/ hia.htm (February 17, 2010).

Chamany, S., L. D. Silver, M. T. Bassett, C. R. Driver, D. K. Berger, C. E. Neuhaus, N. Kumar, and T. R. Frieden. 2009. Tracking diabetes: New York City's A1C registry. *Milbank Quarterly* 87(3):547-570.

City and County of San Francisco Department of Public Health. 2010. *Program on Health, Equity and Sustainability* (October 7, 2010).

Clancy, C. M., and K. Cronin. 2005. Evidence-based decision making: Global evidence, local decisions. *Health Affairs* 24(1):151-162.

Cole, B. L., and J. E. Fielding. 2007. Health impact assessment: A tool to help policy makers understand health beyond health care. *Annual Review of Public Health* 28:393-412.

Cole, B. L., R. Shimkhada, J. E. Fielding, G. Kominski, and H. Morgenstern. 2005. Methodologies for realizing the potential of health impact assessment. *American Journal of Preventive Medicine* 28(4):382-389.

Collins, J. L., J. P. Koplanm, and J. S. Marks. 2009. Chronic disease prevention and control: Coming of age at the Centers for Disease Control and Prevention. *Preventing Chronic Disease Public Health Research, Practice and Policy* 6(3). http://www.cdc.gov/pcd/issues/2009/jul/08_0171.htm (August 20, 2010).

Communities Count. 2008. Introduction. In *Communities Count 2008: Social and Health Indicators Across King County*. Seattle, WA: Communities Count. Pp. ii-4.

Community Health Status Indicators. 2009. *Community Health Status Indicators Report*. http://www.communityhealth.hhs.gov/HomePage.aspx?GeogCD=&PeerStrat=&state=&county= (January 6, 2010).

Congressional Research Service. 2010. *Public Health, Workforce, Quality, and Related Provisions in the Patient Protection and Affordable Care Act (P.L. 111-148)*. Washington, DC: Congressional Research Services.

County Health Rankings. 2010. *How Healthy Is Your County? New County Health Rankings Give First County-by-County Snapshot of Health in Each State*. http://www.countyhealthrankings.org/latest-news/healthday-county-county-report-sizes-americans-health (February 17, 2010).

Dannenberg, A. L., R. Bhatia, B. L. Cole, C. Dora, J. E. Fielding, K. Kraft, D. McClymont-Peace, J. Mindell, C. Onyekere, J. A. Roberts, C. L. Ross, C. D. Rutt, A. Scott-Samuel, and H. H. Tilson. 2006. Growing the field of health impact assessment in the United States: An agenda for research and practice. *American Journal of Public Health* 96(2):262-270.

DeWalt, D. A., N. D. Berkman, S. Sheridan, K. N. Lohr, and M. P. Pignone. 2004. Literacy and health outcomes. *Journal of General Internal Medicine* 19(12):1228-1239.

Doyle, L., and I. Gough. 1991. *A Theory of Human Need*. Hampshire, Bassingstoke: Macmillan.

Drukker, M., S. L. Buka, C. Kaplan, K. McKenzie, and J. Van Os. 2005. Social capital and young adolescents' perceived health in different sociocultural settings. *Social Science & Medicine* 61(1):185-198.

Drummond, M., D. Brixner, M. R. Gold, P. Kind, A. McGuire, and E. Nord. 2009. Toward a consensus on the QALY. *Value in Health* 12(Suppl 1):S31-35.

Epstein, J. M. 2009. Modeling to contain pandemics. *Nature* 460(7256):687-687.

Erickson, P. 1998. Evaluation of a population-based measure of quality of life: The health and activity limitation index (HALex). *Quality of Life Research* 7(2):101-114.

Erickson, P., E. A. Kendall, J. P. Anderson, and R. M. Kaplan. 1989. Using composite health-status measures to assess the nations health. *Medical Care* 27(3):S66-S76.

Evans, R. G., M. L. Barer, and T. R. Marmor, eds. 1990. *Why Are Some People Healthy and Others Not? The Determinants of Health of Populations*. New York: Walter de Gruyter.

Faber, M., M. Bosch, H. Wollersheim, S. Leatherman, and R. Grol. 2009. Public reporting in health care: How do consumers use quality-of-care information? A systematic review. *Medical Care* 47(1):1-8.

Ferrer, M., C. Villasante, J. Alonso, V. Sobradillo, R. Gabriel, G. Vilagut, J. F. Masa, J. L. Viejo, C. A. Jiménez-Ruiz, and M. Miravitlles. 2002. Interpretation of quality of life scores from the St. George's Respiratory Questionnaire. *European Respiratory Journal* 19(3):405-413.

Fisher, E., D. Goodman, J. Skinner, and K. Bronner. 2009. *Health Care Spending, Quality, and Outcomes: More Isn't Always Better*. Lebanon, NH: The Dartmouth Institute for Health Policy and Clinical Practice.

Ford, D., J. Kaufman, and I. Eiron. 2006. An extensible spatial and temporal epidemiological modeling system. *International Journal of Health Geographics* 5(1):4.

Franks, P., P. Muennig, E. Lubetkin, and H. Jia. 2006. The burden of disease associated with being African-American in the United States and the contribution of socio-economic status. *Social Science & Medicine* 62(10):2469-2478.

Friedman, D. J., and R. G. Parrish. 2010. The population health record: Concepts, definition, design, and implementation. *Journal of the American Medical Informatics Association* 17:359-366.

Fryback, D. 2010. *Summary Measures of Population Health: An Overview*. Presentation to the IOM Committee on Public Health Strategies to Improve Health. Washington, DC: IOM.

Fryback, D. G., N. C. Dunham, M. Palta, J. Hanmer, J. Buechner, D. Cherepanov, S. A. Herrington, R. D. Hays, R. M. Kaplan, T. G. Ganiats, D. Feeny, and P. Kind. 2007. U.S. Norms for six generic health-related quality-of-life indexes from the national health measurement study. *Medical Care* 45(12):1162-1170.

Fu, M. C. 2006. Gradient Estimation. In *Handbooks in Operations Research and Management Science*. Vol. 13, edited by G. H. Shane and L. N. Barry. Boston, MA: Elsevier. Pp. 575-616.

Garber, A. M., and H. C. Sox. 2010. The role of costs in comparative effectiveness research. *Health Affairs* 29(10):1805-1811.

Glanz, K. 2009. Measuring food environments: A historical perspective. *American Journal of Preventive Medicine* 36(4):S93-S98.

Gold, M. R., and P. Muennig. 2002. Measure-dependent variation in burden of disease estimates: Implications for policy. *Medical Care* 40(3):260-266.

Gold, M. R., K. I. McCoy, and J. E. Siegel, eds. 1996. *Cost-Effectiveness in Health and Medicine*. New York, NY: Oxford University Press.

Gold, M. R., D. Stevenson, and D. G. Fryback. 2002. HALYS and QALYS and DALYS, oh my: Similarities and differences in summary measures of population health. *Annual Review of Public Health* 23:115-134.

Hammond, R. A. 2008. *A Complex Systems Approach to Understanding and Combating the Obesity Epidemic*. Washington, DC: The Brookings Institution.

Hannon, G. J., and D. Beach. 1994. P15INK4B is a potential effector of TGF-Beta-Induced cell cycle arrest. *Nature* 371(6494):257-261.

Harris, J. 1987. Qalyfying the value of life. *Journal of Medical Ethics* 13(3):117-123.

HHS (Department of Health and Human Services). 2002. *Developing a 21st Century Vision for Health Statistics*. http://www.ncvhs.hhs.gov/21stcent.htm (November 3, 2010).

HHS. 2009a. *Healthy People 2020: Objective Selection Criteria*. http://www.healthypeople.gov/hp2020/objectives/selectionCriteria.aspx (April 28, 2010).

HHS. 2009b. *Secretary's Advisory Committee on National Health Promotion and Disease Prevention Objectives for 2020: Data & IT, Implementation, Evidence-Based Actions, Process for Choosing National Priorities*. http://www.healthypeople.gov/HP2020/Advisory/FACA14Minutes.htm (November 11, 2010).

HHS. 2010. *HHS Gateway to Data and Statistics*. http://www.hhs-stat.net/ (November 15, 2010).

HHS, CDC, and NCHS (National Center for Health Statistics). 2001. *Healthy People 2000: Final Review*. Hyattsville, MD: Public Health Services.

HHS, CDC, and NCVHS (National Committee on Vital and Health Statistics). 2002. *Shaping a Health Statistics Vision for the 21st Century*. Washington, DC: HHS.

Hibbard, J. H., J. Stockard, E. R. Mahoney, and M. Tusler. 2004. Development of the patient activation measure (PAM): Conceptualizing and measuring activation in patients and consumers. *Health Services Research* 39(4p1):1005-1026.

Hibbard, J. H., J. Stockard, and M. Tusler. 2005. Hospital performance reports: Impact on quality, market share, and reputation. *Health Affairs* 24(4):1150-1160.

Hinman, A. R., and D. A. Ross. 2010. Immunization registries can be building blocks for national health information systems. *Health Affairs* 29(4):676-682.

Homer, J., G. Hirsch, and B. Milstein. 2007. Chronic illness in a complex health economy: The perils and promises of downstream and upstream reforms. *System Dynamics Review* 23(2-3):313-343.

Hutton, D. W., D. Tan, S. K. So, and M. L. Brandeau. 2007. Cost-effectiveness of screening and vaccinating Asian and Pacific Islander adults for Hepatitis B. *Annals of Internal Medicine* 147(7):460-469.

IOM (Institute of Medicine). 1998. *Summarizing Population Health: Directions for the Development and Application of Population Metrics.* Washington, DC: National Academy Press.

IOM. 2000. *To Err Is Human: Building a Safer Health System.* Washington, DC: National Academy Press.

IOM. 2003. Assuring America's Health. In *The Future of the Public's Health in the 21st Century.* Washington, DC: The National Academies Press.

IOM. 2004. *Health Literacy: Prescription to End Confusion.* Washington, DC: The National Academies Press.

IOM. 2006. *Performance Measurement: Accelerating Improvement.* Washington, DC: The National Academies Press.

IOM. 2009. *State of the USA Health Indicators: Letter Report.* Washington, DC: The National Academies Press.

IOM. 2010a. Transcript, *Second Meeting of the IOM Committee on Public Health Strategies to Improve Health.* Washington, DC: IOM.

IOM. 2010b. Transcript, *Third Meeting of the IOM Committee on Public Health Strategies to Improve Health.* Washington, DC: IOM.

Jakubowski, B., and H. Frumkin. 2010. Environmental metrics for community health improvement. *Preventing Chronic Disease Public Health Research, Practice and Policy* 7(4). http://www.cdc.gov/pcd/issues/2010/jul/09_0242.htm (July 4, 2010).

Jia, H., and E. I. Lubetkin. 2010. Trends in Quality-Adjusted Life-Years Lost Contributed by Smoking and Obesity. *American Journal of Preventive Medicine* 38(2):138-144.

Kaplan, R. M. 1994. Value judgment in the Oregon Medicaid experiment. *Medical Care* 32(10):975-988.

Kim, Y.-M., and J. A. Neff. 2010. Direct and indirect effects of parental influence upon adolescent alcohol use: A structural equation modeling analysis. *Journal of Child & Adolescent Substance Abuse* 19(3):244-260.

Kizer, K. W., and R. A. Dudley. 2009. Extreme makeover: Transformation of the veterans health care system. *Annual Review of Public Health* 30:313-339.

The Kohala Center. 2008. *Current Events: Hawai'i County Agricultural Development Plan Health Impact Assessment.* http://www.kohalacenter.org/agplan.html (October 7, 2010).

Koivusalo, M. 2010. The state of Health-in-all-Policies (HiAP) in the European Union: Potential and pitfalls. *Journal of Epidemiology and Community Health* 64:500-503.

Kominski, G. F., P. A. Simon, A. Ho, J. Luck, Y. W. Lim, and J. E. Fielding. 2002. Assessing the burden of disease and injury in Los Angeles County using Disability-Adjusted Life Years. *Public Health Reports* 117(2):185-191.

Kominski, G. F., P. A. Simon, A. Y. Ho, and J. E. Fielding. 2010. Financial burdens and disability-adjusted life years in Los Angeles County. In *Handbook of Disease Burdens and Quality of Life Measures,* edited by V. R. Preedy and R. R. Watson. New York: Springer. Pp. 473-482.

Lantz, P. M., and A. Pritchard. 2010. Socioeconomic indicators that matter for population health. *Preventing Chronic Disease Public Health Research, Practice and Policy* 7(4). http://www.cdc.gov/pcd/issues/2010/jul/09_0246.htm (July 4, 2010).

Law, A. M. 2007. *Simulation Modeling and Analysis.* 4th Edition. Boston, MA: McGraw-Hill.

Lowdell, C., M. Bardsley, and D. Morgan. 1999. *Acheson Report: The Inquiry into Inequalities in Health, Implications for London.* London, England: Health of Londoners Project.

Lubetkin, E., H. Jia, P. Franks, and M. Gold. 2005. Relationship among sociodemographic factors, clinical conditions, and health-related quality of life: Examining the EQ-5D in the U.S. general population. *Quality of Life Research* 14(10):2187-2196.

Luck, J., C. Chang, E. R. Brown, and J. Lumpkin. 2006. Using local health information to promote public health. *Health Affairs* 25(4):979-991.

Lytle, L. 2009. Measuring the food environment: State of the science. *American Journal of Preventive Medicine* 36(4): S134 -S144.

Mabry, P. L., S. E. Marcus, P. I. Clark, S. J. Leischow, and D. Mendez. 2010. Systems science: A revolution in public health policy research. *American Journal of Public Health* 100(7):1161-1163.

Madans, J. H. 2008. *The Definition and Measurements of Disability: The Work of the Washington Group.* Presentation to the Washington Group on Disability Statistics. Washington, DC.

Madans, J. H. 2009. *Development of Internationally Comparable Disability Measures: The Washington Group on Disability Statistics.* Presentation to the Washington Group on Disability Statistics. Washington, DC.

Mancuso, C. A., and M. Rincon. 2006. Impact of health literacy on longitudinal asthma outcomes. *Journal of General Internal Medicine* 21(8):813-817.

Mangione, C. M., P. P. Lee, P. R. Gutierrez, K. Spritzer, S. Berry, R. D. Hays, and the National Eye Institute Visual Function Questionnaire Field Test Investigators. 2001. Development of the 25-item National Eye Institute visual function questionnaire. *Archives of Ophthalmology* 119(7):1050-1058.

Manuel, D. G., and S. E. Schultz. 2004. Using linked data to calculate summary measures of population health: Health-adjusted life expectancy of people with diabetes mellitus. *Population Health Metrics* 2(1):4.

The Marmot Review. 2010. *Fair Society, Healthy Lives: Strategic Review of Health Inequalities in England Post-2010.* London, England: The Marmot Review.

Mass, C. F., D. Ovens, K. Westrick, and B. A. Colle. 2002. Does increasing horizontal resolution produce more skillful forecasts? *Bulletin of the American Meteorological Society* 83(3):407-430.

Mayberry, D., and N. Hunkins. 2008. *Health Information Technology (HIT) Report: 2008.* MN: Minnesota Community Measures.

McIntosh, C. N., P. Finès, R. Wilkins, and M. C. Wolfson. 2009. Income disparities in health adjusted life expectancy for Canadian adults, 1991 to 2001. *Statistics Canada* 20(4):1-11.

Meenan, R. F., P. M. Gertman, J. H. Mason, and R. Dunaif. 1982. The Arthritis Impact Measurement Scales: Further investigations of a health status measure. *Arthritis and Rheumatism* 25(9):1048-1053.

Mikkonen, J., and D. Raphael. 2010. *Social Determinants of Health: The Canadian Facts.* Toronto, Canada: York University School of Health Policy and Management.

Milstein, B. 2008. *Hygeia's constellation: Navigating health futures in a dynamic and democratic world.* Atlanta, CA: CDC, Syndemics Prevention Network.

Mitchell, R. J., R. J. McClure, J. Olivier, and W. L. Watson. 2009. Rational allocation of australia's research dollars: Does the distribution of NHMRC funding by national health priority area reflect actual disease burden? *Medical Journal of Australia* 191(11-12):648-652.

Mosen, D., J. Hibbard, and C. Remmers. 2007. Is patient activation associated with outcomes of care for adults with chronic conditions. *Journal of Ambulatory Care Management* 30(1):21-29.

Muennig, P., P. Franks, H. Jiac, E. Lubetkind, and M. R. Gold. 2005. The income-associated burden of disease in the United States. *Social Science and Medicine* 61:2018-2026.

Muennig, P., K. Fiscella, D. Tancredi, and P. Franks. 2010. The relative health burden of selected social and behavioral risk factors in the United States: Implications for policy. *American Journal of Public Health* 100(9):1758-1764.

Murray, C. J., and A. D. Lopez. 2000. Progress and directions in refining the global burden of disease approach: A response to Williams. *Health Economics* 9(1):69-82.

Murray, C. J., J. A. Salomon, and C. Mathers. 2000. A critical examination of summary measures of population health. *Bulletin of the World Health Organization* 78(8):981-994.

Murray, C. J. L., J. A. Salomon, C. D. Mathers, and A. D. Lopez, eds. 2002. *Summary measures of population health: Concepts, ethics, measurement and application.* Geneva, Switzerland: World Health Organization.

National Complete Streets Coalition. 2010. *Complete Streets: FAQ.* http://www.complete streets.org/complete-streets-fundamentals/complete-streets-faq (November 19, 2010).

National Prevention Health Promotion and Public Health Council. 2010. *2010 Annual Status Report.* Washington, DC: HHS.

Navarro-Barrientos, J., D. Rivera, and L. Collins. 2010. A dynamical systems model for understanding behavioral interventions for weight loss. *Advances in Social Computing* 6007:170-179.

NCCOR (National Collaborative on Childhood Obesity Research). 2010. *Envision Project: Using Systems Models to Assess Public Health Policies and Interventions for Childhood Obesity Prevention and Control.* http://www.nccor.org/projects_envision.html (September 8, 2010).

NCHS (National Center for Health Statistics). 2008. *Final Report of the National Health Interview Survey Review Panel to the NCHS Board of Scientific Counselors: Executive Summary.* Atlanta, GA: CDC.

NCHS. 2009. *Report of the NHANES Review Panel to the NCHS Board of Scientific Counselors.* Atlanta, GA: CDC.

NCVHS (National Committee on Vital and Health Statistics). 2008. *Charge of the Subcommittee on Population Health.* http://www.ncvhs.hhs.gov/popschrg.htm (June 17, 2010).

NCVHS. 2010. *Toward Enhanced Information Capacities for Health: An NCVHS Concept Paper.* Washington, DC: HHS.

Neumann, P. J., and D. Greenberg. 2009. Is the United States ready for QALYs? *Health Affairs* 28(5):1366-1371.

Neumann, P. J., and M. C. Weinstein. 2010. Legislating against use of cost-effectivness information. *New England Journal of Medicine* 363(16):1495-1497.

New York City Department of Health and Mental Hygiene. 2009. *Primary Care Information Project.* http://www.nyc.gov/html/doh/html/pcip/pcip.shtml (November 19, 2010).

NORC (National Opinion Research Center). 2005. *Assessment of the Uses and Users of Healthier US and Healthy People 2010.* Washington, DC: NORC.

NRC (National Research Council). 2009. *Principles and Practices for a Federal Statistical Agency.* 4th Edition. Washington, DC: The National Academies Press.

Orszag, P. 2008. *The Overuse, Underuse, and Misuse of Health Care: Testimony Before the Committee on Finance, United States Senate.* Washington, DC: Congressional Budget Office.

Paasche-Orlow, M. K., and M. S. Wolf. 2007. The causal pathways linking health literacy to health outcomes. *American Journal of Health Behavior* 31(Supplement):S19-26.

Pearcy, J. N., and K. G. Keppel. 2002. A summary measure of health disparity. *Public Health Report* 117(3):273-280.

Pearl, J. 2000. *Causality: Models, Reasoning, and Inference.* Cambridge, United Kingdom: Cambridge University Press.

Pearson, S. D., and M. D. Rawlins. 2005. Quality, innovation, and value for money: NICE and the British National Health Service. *Journal of the American Medical Association* 294(20):2618-2622.

Peng, R. D., H. H. Chang, M. L. Bell, A. McDermott, S. L. Zeger, J. M. Samet, and F. Dominici. 2008. Coarse particulate matter air pollution and hospital admissions for cardiovascular and respiratory diseases among Medicare patients. *Journal of the American Medical Association* 299(18):2172-2179.

Pope, C. A., III, M. Ezzati, and D. W. Dockery. 2009. Fine-particulate air pollution and life expectancy in the United States. *New England Journal of Medicine* 360(4):376-386.

Prentice, J. C. 2006. Neighborhood effects on primary care access in Los Angeles. *Social Science and Medicine* 62(5):1291-1303.

Rawles, J. 1989. Castigating QALYs. *Journal of Medical Ethics* 15(3):143-147.

Russell, L. B., M. R. Gold, J. E. Siegel, N. Daniels, and M. C. Weinstein. 1996. The role of cost-effectiveness analysis in health and medicine: Panel on cost-effectiveness in health and medicine. *Journal of the American Medical Association* 276(14):1172-1177.

Safran, C., M. Bloomrosen, W. Hammond, S. Labkoff, S. Markel-Fox, P. C. Tang, and D. E. Detmer. 2007. Toward a national framework for the secondary use of health data: An American Medical Informatics Association white paper. *Journal of the American Medical Informatics Association* 14(1):1-9.

Saskatoon Regional Health Authority. 2007. *2006-2007 Annual Report to the Minister of Health and the Minister of Healthy Living Services.* Saskatoon, Canada: Saskatoon Regional Health Authority.

Schauffler, H. H., and J. K. Mordavsky. 2001. Consumer reports in health care: Do they make a difference? *Annual Review of Public Health* 22:69-89.

Shen, H., and H. Wan. 2009. Controlled sequential factorial design for simulation factor screening. *European Journal of Operational Research* 198(2):511-519.

Statistics Canada. 2010. *Health Models.* http://statcan.gc.ca/microsimulation/health-sante/health-sante-eng.htm (August 26, 2010).

Stiefel, M. C., R. J. Perla, and B. L. Zell. 2010. A healthy bottom line: Healthy life expectancy as an outcome measure for health improvement efforts. *Milbank Quarterly* 88(1):30-53.

Stiglitz, J. E., A. Sen, and J. P. Fitoussi. 2009. *Report by the Commission on the Measurement of Economic Performance and Social Progress.* French Republic: President of the French Republic.

Subramanian, S., G. Bobashev, and R. J. Morris. 2010. When budgets are tight, there are better options than colonoscopies for colorectal cancer screening. *Health Affairs* 29(9):1734-1740.

Taskforce on Health Status. 2005 (November 14-16). *Criteria for and Selection of Domains for the Measurement of Health Status.* Presentation given at the Conference of European Statisticians, Budapest, Hungary.

UCLA HIA-CLIC (Health Impact Assessment-Clearinghouse Learning and Information Center). 2010. *Completed HIAs.* http://www.hiaguide.org/hias?page=1 (August 26, 2010).

The United Nations. 2010 (January). *Brief Historical Overview of the Budapest Initiative and Testing Activities.* Geneva, Switzerland: United Nations Conference.

USDA (United States Department of Agriculture). 2010. *About the Food Environment Atlas.* http://ers.usda.gov/FoodAtlas/about.htm (September 8, 2010).

White House Task Force on Childhood Obesity. 2010. *Solving the Problem of Childhood Obesity Within a Generation.* Washington, DC: Executive Office of the President of the United States.

WHO (World Health Organization). 2010. *Health Impact Assessment.* http://www.who.int/hia/en/ (September 8, 2010).

WHO and ECHP (European Center for Health Policy). 1999. *Health Impact Assessment: Main Concepts and Suggested Approach.* Brussels, Belgium: WHO.

WHO, UNECE (United Nations Economic Commission for Europe), and Eurostat. 2007. *Rationale for the Budapest Initiative-Mark 1 Questionnaire.* Geneva, Switzerland: United Nations Economic Commission for Europe.

Wolfson, M. C. 1999. Measuring health-visions and practicality. *Statistical Journal of the United Nations Economic Commission for Europe* 16:1-17.

Wolfson, M., and G. Rowe. 2009. *Healthpaths Dynamics 2—Using Functional Health Trajectories to Quantify the Sources of Health Inequalities.* Paper presented at International Microsimulation Association 2009, Ottawa, Ontario.

Zhu, X., and C. Lee. 2008. Walkability and safety around elementary schools: Economic and ethnic disparities. *American Journal of Preventive Medicine* 34(4):282-290.

4

Measurement and Accountability

Accountability refers to "the principle that individuals, organizations and the community are responsible for their actions and may be required to explain them to others" (Benjamin et al., 2006). The notion of accountability has several meanings that span the fields of accounting, law, ethics, management theory and practice, and governance. Models of accountability include regulatory, legal, accreditation or certification (sometimes quasiregulatory), and pay-for-performance models, or their public health equivalent, eligibility for funding based on past performance. This chapter does not endeavor to examine all dimensions of accountability but rather focuses on the role of indicators in holding to account all stakeholders that contribute to the conditions for health in a community. Other dimensions of accountability will be examined in the committee's later reports on public health law and funding. Two important examples are the intertwined topics of political will and governance (and governing bodies).[1] As noted in this chapter, the governance (and related regulatory and funding) mechanisms that pertain to the work of local public health agencies are among the stronger and more concrete levers for holding agencies accountable.

This chapter examines performance[2] indicators and how they can be implemented both at the level of governmental public health and in the con-

---

[1] The National Public Health Performance Standards Program defines *governing body* as "the individual, board, council, commission, or other body with legal authority over the primary governmental public health agency" (HHS and CDC, 2008).

[2] *Performance* refers to the interventions—policies, programs, and processes—implemented with the intent of improving population health; it represents one of the steps along the inputs-to-outputs or inputs-to-outcomes logic model presented in Chapter 2.

tributions of other health-system stakeholders. (As defined in Chapter 1, the health system comprises public health, clinical care, and other stakeholders that acknowledge their current and potential contributions to a community's health.)

Governmental public health is not the only actor in the system that is accountable for or involved in creating the conditions for health. Clinical care providers are de facto stewards of a community's health and are mandated or otherwise charged with health-related duties. Others, such as employers and businesses, may not currently see themselves as contributing to or detracting from a community's health and well-being (see Chapter 1), but their recognition of their roles and their ability to contribute to health could be facilitated. They often face regulatory pressures, such as rules regarding environmental waste and pollution and zoning limitations. Others, such as community-based organizations, may be seasoned contributors to health, but there are no measurement frameworks for accountability for their work. Those roles are discussed in greater detail later in this chapter.

The measurement of performance and the demonstration of accountability and quality in clinical care have a long history, with a major national movement punctuated by milestone Institute of Medicine (IOM) reports on the subject of quality, federal quality initiatives (such as those undertaken by the Centers for Medicaid and Medicare Services), and the creation of such bodies as the National Committee for Quality Assurance (and its Healthcare Effectiveness Data and Information Set quality measures) and the National Quality Forum and its efforts to set national priorities and endorse standards for and conduct outreach and education on performance improvement in clinical care.

Accountability (in the broad sense of demonstrating results and effectiveness to the public) is a somewhat more recent focus in the public health community, and this is in part due to the complex array of factors that contribute to population health and the challenging nature of communicating about them. As described in Chapter 1, one challenge is that health outcomes (such as disease and death) have multiple interconnected causal pathways, and the science required to elucidate them is far from advanced in many cases. In addition, public health agencies, although broadly charged with ensuring the public's health, have direct or clearly traceable responsibility for only a small proportion of those pathways.

The simple logic model introduced in Chapter 2 and reprised in Figure 4-1 suggests that a straightforward measurement framework for accountability would link all inputs (resources, capacities, processes, interventions, and policies) with outputs (intermediate and more distal health outcomes). However, there are many obstacles to such a framework, and these are discussed below. It is important to note that accountability is closely linked with needs assessment, planning, and priority-setting—activities identified at the beginning of the process.

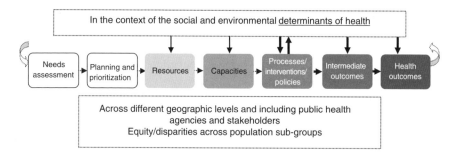

FIGURE 4-1 From inputs to outputs logic model.
NOTE: The thickness of some arrows denotes the present report's focus on those interactions.

The committee recognizes that detailed performance objectives may be identified and measurements conducted at each step of the continuum depicted in Figure 4-1 by all stakeholders in the system. For example, there may be specific objectives for public health agencies or for hospitals that assess their community's health needs, objectives for the process of planning (such as the number of partners engaged in planning and collaborative planning activities undertaken), objectives that monitor resource use, and so on. In this chapter, however, the committee focuses on the "macro" or broader accountability for the entire continuum of community-health improvement (from needs assessment to the most distal outcomes) and not on any detail of the "micro" accountabilities that could be examined and described for each step in the process.

In the process of community-health improvement, after a community's health needs are assessed, priorities are identified, and plans are made and implemented, performance measurement is needed to hold implementers (the full spectrum of system stakeholders in addition to public health agencies) accountable and to spur continuous quality improvement to increase the effectiveness, efficiency, and equity of actions taken to improve population health. Performance measurement is the main way to monitor accountability in the health system.

A FRAMEWORK FOR ACCOUNTABILITY

The measurement framework for accountability discussed in this chapter applies to the delivery of funded public health programs by public health agencies; the role of public health agencies in mobilizing the overall public health system; and the roles, contributions, and performance of health-system partners (other governmental agencies, private-sector stakeholders, and communities).

Assessing and measuring accountability at any level (local, state, or national) and holding organizations accountable require the following four elements:

- An identified body with a clear charge to accomplish particular steps toward health goals.
- Ensuring that the body has the capacity to undertake the required activities.
- Measuring what is accomplished against the identified body's clear charge.
- The availability of tools to assess and improve effectiveness and quality (such as a feedback loop as part of a learning system, incentives, and technical assistance).

Those who influence population health can be held accountable through two models:

- *Contract model:* When an oversight party has direct control over implementers (for example, through statute or funding), standard direct methods of accountability can be used, with the caveat that accountability indicators are used to measure execution of agreed-on strategy. Holding implementers accountable in this context may involve regular programmatic progress reports, such evaluations as program reviews, and other tools typically used in the work of continuous quality improvement.
- *Mutual accountability[3] (or compact) model:* When no oversight party has financial or other direct authority over those who are implementing, stakeholders must assume both an oversight role and an implementation role. Involved parties agree on overall priorities and strategies and then on actions and measures of actions that each organization will undertake. The group—which may take the form of a coalition, alliance, board, or other structure—holds individual organizations accountable for performance through public reporting and other agreed-on mechanisms, such as incentives for future leadership roles and funding. *Compact* refers loosely both to the social compact and to the coalitions or other structures formed in many communities, agreements entered into, and other creative and innovative mechanisms used around the country to bring varied stakeholders together to assess health (or other community needs), devise strategies for improving it, and evaluate performance in

---

[3] *Mutual accountability* is used in international-development circles (for example, OECD, 2009; World Bank, 2008). OECD (2009) defines it as "a process by which partners hold one another responsible for the commitments that they have voluntarily made to each other."

implementing the strategies. Frameworks and measures that link interventions to outcomes can help facilitate all this.

For example, in contract accountability, funds might be given to a stakeholder by local government or by a foundation to create an antitobacco media campaign or by a health department to a community-based organization for provision of smoking-cessation services. In mutual accountability, an agreement might be drafted by an antismoking coalition to advocate jointly for a specific legislative strategy, such as tobacco taxes. In short, the type of accountability depends not on the category of entity but on what it is accountable for doing. Those in the contract model can be held accountable by the individuals, agencies, or organizations that hold authority—legislators, a chief executive, boards of health, public health agencies, a philanthropic organization, taxpayers, and so on. Those who entered into an agreement in the mutual accountability or compact model will be accountable to whomever they have entered into agreement with, possibly including an array of system stakeholders.

This framework for accountability works whether or not the oversight party has financial, administrative, or other control over the implementing party, but the specifics must be operationalized differently in the two settings. Regardless of setting, accountability depends on good measurement and links to the standard sets of outcome measures and measures of community health in Chapter 3, Recommendation 2. For an overview of the framework for measurement in accountability that the committee discusses in this chapter, see Figure 4-2. An important element of the framework is that health-system partners need to align and coordinate their efforts consistently to ensure the greatest impact and achieve population health goals.

Challenges for Measurement and Accountability

There are many challenges to implementing a measurement framework for accountability. For many of the determinants of health, no specific entity or body is charged with improving a given determinant and made accountable for it. For example, food deserts may be one factor contributing to poor nutritional status and obesity of some Americans (Franco et al., 2009; USDA, 2010), but the authority (or responsibility) for addressing this problem is unclear and widely distributed among various public-sector and private-sector entities (as examples of the former, local government planning and zoning policies, and tax incentives for businesses; and as an example of the latter, supermarket-chain decisions about the location of new stores).

A simple, quantifiable outcome-based measure would be ideal (for example, easy to communicate and easy to understand) for evaluating the performance of public health agencies and other stakeholders in the health

---

BOX 4-1
Evidence Base and Public Health Research

Performance measurement is especially important when evidence to elucidate the pathways from system inputs (such as resources and capacities) to system outputs and outcomes is unavailable. To affect intermediate and ultimate health outcomes (for example, decreases in obesity and in all distal outcomes for which obesity is a primary risk factor, such as diabetes and CVD morbidity and mortality), public health agencies and other stakeholders must use evidence-based population-level interventions whenever possible and translate them into metrics for accountability. Gaps in knowledge should stimulate research and evaluations (Glasgow, 2010).

Individual and population-based strategies (that is, the medical model and the ecologic model) differ considerably, as discussed in Chapter 1. For example, administering a vaccine to a patient is an individual-based intervention; ensuring optimal levels of immunization in a community or nation is a population-based strategy. In many areas, population-based strategies are not well developed and have less precise effect sizes. The nation's public health research enterprise is producing an expanding body of evidence concerning population-level (public health) interventions, programs, and policies that are efficacious and cost-effective in reducing health risks for specific populations at risk (for example, preventive interventions documented in the Guide to Community Preventive Services, 2010).

Many of the interventions have been evaluated for their effects on individual-level health outcomes or outcomes observed in small and controlled population groups. As a result, relatively little evidence suggests what scale of implementation must be achieved to produce a sustained effect on population health at the level of an entire community, region, or state. For example, some evidence suggests the vaccination coverage that needs to be achieved to provide optimal protection against vaccine-preventable diseases, but this type of evidence is lacking for many other types of public health programs, policies, and interventions, such as those which target obesity-prevention programming and food-safety inspection.

Similarly, there is relatively little evidence to suggest how to achieve the scale and quality of implementation needed to affect health on a population

---

system. However, holding the agencies and organizations accountable for specific health outcomes—such as reduced rates of cardiovascular disease (CVD), diabetes, or obesity—or specific modifiable determinants of health, such as smoking prevalence in the community, is not possible for several reasons:

- There is a naturally shifting baseline of diseases and other conditions (both up and down) for all health outcomes in a community, regardless of whether a public health intervention has been implemented.

level. Implementation research at the level of the public health delivery system is needed to produce such evidence, including how best to divide and coordinate implementation responsibilities among available public-sector and private-sector stakeholders and specifically what roles government public health agencies should play vis-à-vis other stakeholders in the health system; what levels of human, monetary, institutional, technologic, and information resources are required for successful implementation; and what complementary mix of services, programs, and activities must be available (for example, enhanced HIV screening will have minimal public health effect if access to treatment is not simultaneously ensured).

There are also large evidence gaps concerning the crosscutting public health practices that are required to facilitate decision-making and to ensure successful implementation of interventions. Those practices include community health assessment, epidemiologic investigation, community health planning, policy development, communication, workforce development, evaluation and monitoring, and quality improvement.

For the public health interventions, programs, and policies that currently are supported by strong evidence, a measurement system is needed to assess adoption, reach, and implementation fidelity at state and local levels. The system would facilitate research to address current gaps in evidence and would support accountability mechanisms. It could also allow detection of practice variation among public health agencies, communities, and states and identify outcomes (health and economic consequences) that result from practice variation, thus allowing targeted improvement in efficiency and effectiveness. Correspondingly, such a system could be used to support public reporting and benchmarking, accreditation and quality-improvement applications, performance-based contracting, and pay-for-performance applications.

There is a lack of precision with which public health workers can say they have achieved outcomes in a given community. The circumstances and programs that maximize health are many, and their relationships with one another are not always well understood. Dynamic models to which information can be added (as described in Chapter 3) can also create an evidence base from which to link salutary processes that lead to better intermediate outcomes that in turn increase the health-adjusted life expectancy of a population.

- There is a lack of precision of the effect size for known interventions—even for those considered best practices—partly because of other underlying conditions in a community (the determinants of health from the individual level of genes to the broadest environmental factors) (see Box 4-1 on evidence-based research).
- There may be stakeholders (such as private-sector entities) that are not part of a framework for accountability whose actions (both supportive of and detrimental to health) can substantially influence the success of interventions.
- There is a lack of knowledge about effective interventions for many health challenges that are identified as priorities. This may require

innovation and implementation of "promising practices" whose efficacy is uncertain (see Box 4-1).

- It may take many years or even decades for the results of public health interventions to materialize. Such long timelines may not meet the needs of policy-makers and the public, who need to see and use intermediate measures that demonstrate progress.

Measuring health outcomes is important and helps the system (at all levels) to know where it stands; owing to the factors listed above, however, distal health outcomes (such as death and diseases) are not useful in the context of accountability. Because of those factors, there is confusion and inconsistency regarding how to implement a framework for accountability in the nation's health system (again, defined as the multiple partners working to improve population health). The lack of such a framework and the lack of consistency (for example, in what is measured) can confuse policy-makers and the public and erode their confidence in system performance. Transparency in measuring performance and in demonstration of accountability to the public and to policy-makers is a critical underpinning of any population health effort.

The committee concludes that a framework for accountability is needed that includes

- Agreement among implementing agencies, stakeholders, and those holding them accountable on specific plans of action for targeting health priorities.
- Holding of implementing agencies or stakeholders accountable for execution of the agreed-on plans (strategies, interventions, policies, and processes).
- Measurement of execution and outcomes of the agreed-on plans and agreement on revisions to a plan of action.

A model of accountability is needed that works both when there are areas with established (for example, evidence-based) best practices (as in the case of tobacco prevention) and when there is a less well-developed evidence base (as in the case of obesity prevention). The framework that the committee proposes applies in both situations because accountability measures assess the execution of agreed-on strategies. In settings where there are best practices based on evidence, accountability is primarily fidelity to established models of effective interventions. In settings where there are no clear best practices, accountability is based primarily on efficient and effective management of agreed-on innovative interventions (or programs or processes), including the placing of a higher premium on evaluation and modification as new information becomes available.

In the larger context of accountability, there are other unique challenges and issues in establishing accountability for population health, including how to align missions of diverse organizations or stakeholders in pursuit of shared population health goals at the environmental level; the need for strategic agreement established through a spectrum of mechanisms, such as law, financial and other types of incentives, and voluntary agreements; addressing challenges inherent in collective action (for example, free riders, or interested parties that benefit but do not contribute); and the presence of internal accountabilities (organization missions) and external accountabilities (contracts, and legal, financial, or social compacts or pressures) throughout the system.

Role of Measurement in Accountability

Measurement has unique and powerful roles to play in an accountability system, especially when other legal and financial drivers of accountability are weak or absent. Measurement can elucidate shared responsibilities for population outcomes and reveal the levels of effort and achievement needed to reach shared objectives. Measurement can be used in tandem with and is also a vehicle for legal mechanisms (such as contract compliance and liability) and incentive and financing mechanisms (such as pay-for-performance, eligibility, and resource allocation).

Measurement comes into play both at the beginning of the accountability process (for example, to inform a community and help it to decide where resources should be directed) and at the end after coordination and development of a strategy and its execution (for example, to measure outcomes of processes of a health department or business). Measurement provides a basis of alignment of efforts among health-system stakeholders. Efforts may be strategies required by law, or agreed on in contracts or agreements. Measuring and reporting on process indicators can help to strengthen accountability pathways. Having indicators available for those who take part in the accountability process may demonstrate the need for greater involvement of all stakeholders in the health system. Indicators could help to illustrate the lack of collective action in the current system in which many of those who can and do affect health (both favorably and adversely) are not part of a formal or organized system. These measures would make the contributions (or lack thereof) of various stakeholders observable and help to spur collective action. The committee's next report will address the legal mechanisms that can assist in the alignment of strategies.

Figure 4-2 depicts a framework for the measurement dimension of accountability that draws on the work of the IOM Committee on Quality of Health Care in America (see Berwick, 2002; IOM, 2001). In that context, a framework was provided to demonstrate the changes needed in the US

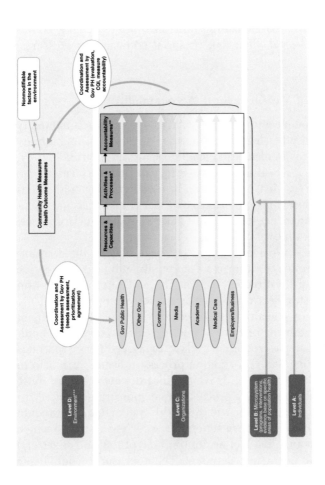

FIGURE 4-2 A framework for measurement in accountability.

NOTE: Gov = Government; PH = Public Health; CQI = Continuous Quality Improvement.

* Activities and processes are influenced by agreed-on strategies (strategies agreed on by those being held accountable and those holding other parties accountable through contracts or compact agreements).

** Accountability measures assess how well the agreed-on strategies are executed and this may also be thought of as strategy execution measures.

***Stakeholder activities both influence the environment and work within it to shape outcomes.

SOURCE: Adapted from Berwick, 2002; IOM, 2001.

medical care delivery system, and four levels were described: Level A, the experience of patients and communities; Level B, the microsystem of care (for example, provider practices); Level C, organizations (for example, managed-care organizations); and Level D, the environment shaped by policy, payment, regulation, and accreditation.

The present committee believes that that framework holds relevance for its own examination of measurement in the context of accountability and has adapted it for its own purposes. The cycle begins after a needs assessment has been done, priorities set, and a plan agreed on. Level A in the committee's adaptation of the framework includes persons (whose aggregated health information constitutes health-outcome measures) and neighborhoods. Level B refers to microsystems, which in the context of population health[4] are programs, policies, and interventions that may be thought to refer to the points of contact or interactions among community groups, local businesses, others in the neighborhood, and their local public health agencies and allied entities. An example of microsystems is an interaction among a health department, a local medical care provider, community coalition, or local business concerning a particular health outcome. Specifically, a health department could assist a food retailer in facilitating healthful customer choices or could support a local business in developing a workplace prevention and wellness program. Often in public health, such microsystems need to align and integrate across organizations; for example, the local cancer-control program should feed into the statewide cancer-control program, which feeds into the national program. Level C consists of organizations described as actors in the public health system in the 2003 IOM report *The Future of the Public's Health in the 21st Century* (IOM, 2003a) and as components of the health system. The organizations include the local public health agency, hospitals and other clinical care entities, community organizations, schools, businesses, religious congregations, and many others that perform roles that influence health outcomes. Level D refers to the environment, which includes a variety of social, physical (both naturally occurring and constructed), and economic factors and is shaped in part by social realities, large-scale policies (and political will), and economic arrangements (Syme and Ritterman, 2009). Figure 4-2 also depicts accountability pathways for all levels but focuses on Level C—the organizations that perform functions that affect health outcomes.

CONTEXT AND HISTORY

Performance measurement and reporting are not new ideas in public health; agencies have had to report on their performance to federal or

---

[4] As is sometimes pointed out, the patient in public health practice is the community.

state funders and to government executives, and a performance-standards movement has been facilitated by the National Public Health Performance Standards (begun by the Centers for Disease Control and Prevention in 1998) and by the Turning Point Performance Management Collaborative (supported by the Robert Wood Johnson Foundation from 1997 to 2001) (NACCHO, 2009a,b; RWJF and W.K. Kellogg Foundation, 2006). Public health agencies also have a long history of planning and evaluation, facilitated by such tools as the National Association of County and City Health Officials *Mobilizing for Action through Planning and Partnerships* framework and the IOM-developed Community Health Improvement Process (IOM, 1997; University of Wisconsin Population Health Institute, 2010). However, broader notions of accountability in public health, especially with regard to the roles of other stakeholders in the system, have arisen more recently.

Accreditation is one mechanism for demonstrating accountability to policy-makers, elected officials, and the community regarding the quality of public health services. The 2003 IOM report *The Future of the Public's Health in the 21st Century* (IOM, 2003a) strongly recommended that public health practice organizations and funders jointly explore the potential of a voluntary accreditation system to improve public health practice performance and demonstrate agency accountability. The recommendation led to the formation of the Exploring Accreditation Project, which found that accreditation was both feasible and desirable as a means of enhancing public health quality improvement efforts and strengthening accountability. As a result, the Public Health Accreditation Board (PHAB) was founded in 2007 and tasked with the development and implementation of the nascent voluntary accreditation system (PHAB, 2009). As expected, given the early stage of development, the current accreditation standards focus primarily on capacity and process measures. In fall 2010, the PHAB completed 30 site visits as part of beta testing of national accreditation standards and measures that will allow public health agencies to be assessed against consensus benchmarks (PHAB, 2010). Future iterations of the standards are expected to also include intermediate and distal health outcome measures. The committee recognizes the importance of objective third-party oversight of the accountability system. As the PHAB evolves, it may provide one option for implementation of an accountability system and framework.

Although there is a considerable history of activity regarding accountability in the context of public health practice, few efforts have been undertaken to develop a measurement framework for accountability in creating population health. Some of the discussion below endeavors to provide guidance in moving forward in this direction.

ROLES OF SYSTEM STAKEHOLDERS IN
MEASURING ACCOUNTABILITY

In this section, the committee discusses how the measurement framework for accountability outlined in this chapter applies in three contexts—(1) nongovernment and private-sector stakeholders, (2) government agencies other than public health agencies, and (3) public health agencies—and makes a recommendation that applies to the entire system, although its implementation and relevant tools may differ somewhat in each context.

Accountability of Nongovernment and Private-Sector Stakeholders

Measuring accountability of nongovernmental or private-sector stakeholders is the most challenging for framing a discussion of accountability because there are few bases for holding them accountable for actions on health, such as statutes or funding. Exceptions include government regulation of private-sector land use and generation of environmental hazards, such as pollutants, but these do not always originate in government concerns about health. However, it is encouraging that multiple stakeholders at the national, state, or local level have acknowledged in recent years that health is the product of collective effort and have thus offered a basis for a type of shared accountability. In most cases, unless funding is provided or other contractual agreements are entered into, these stakeholders will be part of a mutual accountability relationship.

Collaborative efforts with public health agencies and others can support these stakeholders for example, through the preparation of regular reports on the state of a community's health to inform stakeholders and help them to measure their progress. Part of the role of governmental public health agencies is to understand the effectiveness, cost, and outcomes of public health services delivered by all stakeholders; these characteristics could be included in assessing the performance of other actors. Government public health agencies can serve as conveners and facilitators on strategy and tactics and on commitments to collective and individual action by stakeholders. Government public health agencies can also serve as managers or facilitators of incentives that both reward and serve as a tool for holding stakeholders accountable (i.e., driving other sectors to demonstrate accountability on contributions to health improvement), in some cases on behalf of the community in general or a community group. Examples of incentives may be small amounts of funding to community-based organizations, public recognition, special status in competing for government funding, or letters of support to endorse an organization's grant fund-raising efforts.

However, forms of the contract model of accountability may also apply to stakeholders in cases in which government develops incentives or disincentives for businesses or begins a contract with them for various types of

---

BOX 4-2
The Ten Essential Public Health Services

1. **Monitor** health status to identify community health problems.
2. **Diagnose and investigate** health problems and health hazards in the community.
3. **Inform, educate, and empower** people about health issues.
4. **Mobilize** community partnerships to identify and solve health problems.
5. **Develop policies and plans** that support individual and community health efforts.
6. **Enforce** laws and regulations that protect health and ensure safety.
7. **Link** people to needed personal health services and assure the provision of medical care when otherwise unavailable.
8. **Assure** a competent public health and personal healthcare workforce.
9. **Evaluate** effectiveness, accessibility, and quality of personal and population-based health services.
10. **Research** for new insights and innovative solutions to health problems.

SOURCE: Public Health Functions Steering Committee, 1994.

---

work. For example, employers could receive tax advantages for enacting policies and adopting workplace programs and strategies that promote employee health (such as better health plans and at-work programs) (Baicker et al., 2010; Bourgeois et al., 2008; Goetzel and Ozminkowski, 2008; Heinen and Darling, 2009; Houle and Siegel, 2009; Okie, 2007; Ozminkowski et al., 2002).[5] A recent example of the use of tax benefits is found in New York City's FRESH program and in the state of Michigan, both of which offer property-tax incentives for some types of retail food establishments, such as grocery stores (Michigan Department of Community Health, 2008a; NYC Department of City Planning, 2010).

Public health agencies could track and report on these types of contributions to the greater health of a community. Although the "Ten Essential Public Health Services" (see Box 4-2) are often embedded in a statutory

---

[5] A recent literature review by Baicker et al. (2010) showed that employer-based wellness programs have increased substantially, from 19 percent in 2006 to 77 percent in 2008 among employers that have 500 or more employees. The study also found that for every dollar spent on employee wellness programs, there were about $3 in savings, both in medical costs and in absenteeism. In addition, some companies—such as General Mills, Texas Instruments, and Johnson & Johnson—have invested in wellness programs that address obesity, weight loss, disease prevention and management in the workplace, and creating a work culture and environment that support healthy choices that lead to healthy behavior (Heinen and Darling, 2009; Ozminkowski et al., 2002).

context and represent the fundamental roles of public health agencies (Public Health Functions Steering Committee, 1994), others in communities can contribute to some of the services. That is especially true of medical care organizations, particularly those with large community presences and wide portfolios of community-benefit (such as health-promotion) activities. With the enactment of the Affordable Care Act (ACA), the role of public health agencies in providing safety-net medical care services (part of Essential Public Health Service 7; see Box 4-2) and their relationship with the publicly and privately funded clinical care system may change dramatically. Although it was outside the scope of the present committee's task to specify how public health agencies should change after implementation of the ACA, the committee recognizes the potential benefits and some challenges that may emerge from the expansion of medical insurance. (The committee may gather information on the evolution of these issues in preparing its future reports on public health law and resources.)

Accountability of Government Agencies

The 2003 IOM report *The Future of the Public's Health in the 21st Century* did not explicitly identify government agencies other than public health agencies as contributors to the health system, but it did refer to education, transportation, and other factors that contribute to health outcomes and that "reside" in other sectors of government (IOM, 2003b). In recent years, there have been efforts across the country to examine the ramifications of all types of policy decisions on health outcomes by using such tools as health impact assessments as part of an approach, also used internationally, called Health in All Policies (CDC, 2010; Koivusalo, 2010). As described in Chapter 3, a recent example is the National Prevention, Health Promotion, and Public Health Council, which comprises many department and agency heads under the leadership of the surgeon general of the Public Health Service. Government agencies charged with planning, transportation, education, and other civic functions have begun to consider the synergistic effects of multiple factors that create health in a community, and evidence is being amassed to demonstrate the mutual benefits of considering health effects as part of other types of planning, design, and tracking processes. Several government agencies outside the Department of Health and Human Services (HHS) and the state and local public health agencies are charged with addressing health issues—for example, the US Department of Agriculture and the Environmental Protection Agency (EPA) at the federal level—and other agencies without overt health-related duties (such as local planning departments) represent the government as well and therefore have a duty to contribute to the implementation policies and programs that serve the larger public good, of which health is both a foundation and a component.

BOX 4-3
Examples of Actual or Potential Synergy
Among Government Sectors in the
Improvement of Population Health

Many communities have found that planners and epidemiologists (among many others) can collaborate on issues of mutual interest, such as design and infrastructure features of cities and suburbs that support health objectives. For example, recent research suggests that some types of public transportation increase the physical activity of community residents and have the potential to lead to improvement in multiple health outcomes (MacDonald et al., 2010).

San Francisco's departments of public health and of housing have worked collaboratively to rebuild and transform living conditions in three public-housing sites (for more information, see The Healthy Development Measurement Tool, 2006). For an example of evidence on the relevance of housing to health outcomes, see Krieger and Higgins (2002) and Keall et al. (2010).

To reduce high infant mortality, Detroit's health department has worked with other parts of local government to improve the services and supports available to pregnant women and has thus transformed the social and economic environmental factors partly responsible for poor outcomes (Michigan Department of Community Health, 2008b).

Local government agencies, from education to planning to transportation, have roles in supporting and improving quality of life and facilitating some aspects of social progress. However, the effects of other government sectors on population health have been largely invisible to the agencies (whether at the national, state, or local level), in part because of the medical care focus of the nation, policy-makers, and the public. The discussions in Chapter 2 and 3 illustrate the potential contributions of measurement to informing other sectors about how they affect population health outcomes favorably or unfavorably. Box 4-3 provides some examples of potential or actual kinds of collaboration among government sectors, including public health.

The American public and nonprofit sectors increasingly recognize that most parts of government—whether at the national, state, or local level—can contribute to improvements in health and that health is closely intertwined with income and economic opportunity, education, housing, and other factors (see Chapter 2 for a discussion of determinants of health). Such recent efforts as the Department of Education's Promise Neighborhoods; the First Lady's "Let's Move!" Campaign with its attention to food deserts in vulnerable communities (White House Task Force on Childhood Obesity, 2010); the Interagency Partnership for Sustainable Communities of the Department of Transportation (DOT), the Department of Housing and Urban Development (HUD), and EPA (National Center for Appropriate Technology, 2010); and the exploration of opportunities for collaboration at the intersection of health and community development by the Robert Wood Johnson Foundation and the Federal Reserve (Syme and Ritterman, 2009) are among the higher-profile examples of intersectoral collaborative efforts to improve health and its determinants. One of the principles of the DOT, HUD, and EPA partnership is valuing communities and neighborhoods by "enhanc[ing] the unique characteristics of all communities by investing in healthy, safe, and walkable neighborhoods" (EPA, 2010).

Federal partnerships to address aspects of community well-being that include or contribute to health signal federal-government interest in supporting similar interactions in communities at all levels and model the possibilities for similar collaborations at the local level. However, many communities already have a strong record of collaborative efforts to improve health that commonly are facilitated or convened by a local public health agency. Many of the local-level indicator sets that the committee reviewed (some are provided as examples in Appendix B) are tools used by such communities as Seattle–King County, Alameda County in California, and Saskatoon, Canada (Alameda County Public Health Department, 2008; Lemstra and Neudorf, 2008; Seattle and King County Public Health Department, 2010). Reports prepared by such communities highlight diverse partnerships that include agencies of the local government. However, many of the reports and measurement tools largely reflect health outcomes and to a far smaller extent the determinants of health in a given community. The indicator sets do not attempt to link performance of other government agencies (or other stakeholders) to the outcomes reported; this is understandable, given the challenges described in this chapter. However, the committee believes that demonstrating accountability is essential and that developing meaningful, valid, and fair measures of accountability for public-sector agencies other than public health agencies is important and reasonably achievable in light of the agencies' own responsibilities for community well-being (and the potential for synergistic effects of collaboration of the community with public health agencies) and public health agencies' proven ability to inform, mobilize, and convene. Tools to facilitate shared ("compact") accountability to communities may include joint reporting by public health and other relevant agencies on issues of mutual interest that influence the health of constituents in a jurisdiction. Other government agencies may be subject to the same kind of accountability as public health agencies to the extent that federal, state, and local funds are linked to specific strategies or to the chief elected official to whom they report on mandated activities (contract accountability). A recommendation and sample accountability measures are provided at the end of this chapter.

Public Health Agency Accountability

Accountability is typically linked to specific statutory authority, fiduciary duty, obligation to demonstrate return on investment, or other formal relationships. This may be called contract accountability. This type of accountability clearly characterizes government public health agencies (as opposed to other government agencies or private sector entities)—at local, state, and federal levels—that hold primary responsibility for the health of their population or community (see Box 4-2 for a list of the Ten Essential Public Health Services). Public health agencies may also be part of compact- or mutual accountability arrangements, discussed later.

In addition to their own accountability for discharging their statutory duties and using federal, state, and local funding appropriately, public health agencies are stewards of a community's overall health and can play the role of monitors, conveners, or rapporteurs with respect to the performance and accomplishments of other stakeholders in the health system. Public health agencies can also cultivate collaborative relationships with other government agencies by explaining how coordinated efforts that make use of the opportunities afforded by different entities can have health benefits that spill over into other sectors that will continue to build the overall health and quality of life of a community.

Public health agencies play several major roles with implications for accountability. They deliver funded public health programs that include traditional activities such as sanitation and food safety and some safety-net clinical care services, and they have the potential to and often do mobilize or convene the overall health system in a community to transform the conditions for health. The level of accountability of public health agencies is based partly on their capacity, size, and resources. As agencies change their plans in response to a changing environment, including reforms in insurance and the provision of medical care triggered by the ACA (HHS, 2010), public health programs, budgets, and funding streams will also require change. This will be addressed in greater detail in the committee's third report, on funding for public health. The committee notes that some legacy programs remain necessary and does not recommend wholesale dismantling of the existing system of funding and programs, but some level of reallocation will be needed. In addition, accountabilities will probably vary by community, and their foci, specific activities, and expenditures will probably not be amenable to a uniform set of metrics, but outlining some common criteria will be useful.

The role of public health agencies is to ensure "the conditions in which people can be healthy" (IOM, 1988, 2003a). As the nature and the understanding of preventable death and disability have changed (as discussed in Chapter 1), the information available to public health agencies has suggested a need to change priorities and strategies. Although public health agencies rightly seek to sustain past achievements—such as successes over infectious diseases and improvements in maternal and child health and tobacco control and dependence—they are also called on to respond to emerging challenges to population health, such as obesity and injury. For example, they can develop or select new tools (such as policy changes), nurture new relationships and alliances, and restructure existing programs and structures to maximize available resources.

There are several challenges to the ability of the public health infrastructure to address high-priority population health concerns effectively and efficiently. Challenges include a mismatch between the targets of public health funding and resources and the leading causes of preventable deaths and illnesses (an issue the committee intends to address more fully in its later report on funding). There is a skills mismatch in which public health practice might not match current or emerging challenges (including infectious disease), and there is a great need to strengthen skills and capacity to interact with and influence such spheres as policy systems and the environment (for example, with place-based changes). Finally, interventions to address emerging problems, such as obesity, are far from having gathered the strength of evidence that characterizes infectious-disease control, tobacco use, or some aspects of vehicle safety, and the legislative or statutory basis of such interventions is in its infancy. For example, before the passage of the ACA (with its provision requiring calorie-posting and other nutritional disclosures beyond some threshold by some restaurant, food-outlet, and vending-machine businesses), a small number of jurisdictions had enacted laws that require all restaurants to post some types of nutritional information (NPLAN, 2009; Simon et al., 2008). In the absence of such laws pertaining to nutrition or other issues (it should be noted that the national law does not pertain to smaller businesses, such as ones that have fewer than 20 retail sites), public health agencies must rely on other tools, such as their influence and collaboration with community partnerships to facilitate change. (The legal context of population health improvement will be discussed in a later report.) On the one hand, the status of many legal interventions is complicated by the fact that the effectiveness of such laws in modifying behaviors is not established; on the other hand, it seems imperative that public health agencies use the best available evidence and undertake innovations that may yield results and advance the evidence base. Developing measures of accountability based on guaranteed specific quantifiable changes in health outcomes would be particularly problematic in areas where the evidence is incomplete, and the measurement framework for accountability proposed by the committee in this report may provide a needed alternative. The broadest (or most upstream) determinants of health—such as poverty, education, and disparities resulting from discrimination—have relevance to the work of public health agencies, but they require broad-based partnerships and mobilization of communities to change norms or values regarding what a community finds and does not find acceptable among the fundamental determinants of health. A further challenge is that many of the interventions lie outside even the most generous assessment of a public health skill set, and the nature of effective interventions remains very elusive.

Public health agencies are held accountable in a variety of ways: directly to funders, heads of the executive branch, and boards of health where applicable, and indirectly to the communities they serve (see, for example, Alameda County Public Health Department, 2008; Communities Count, 2008; Department of Population Health Sciences, 2008; Office of Health Assessment and Epidemiology, 2010; Summers et al., 2009). Many public health agencies track and describe their use of resources and performance in a variety of formats, including progress reports to federal, state, and local funders and annual reports to the public, such as citizens of a county or city. In its environmental-health role, public health agencies are held accountable with process measures (such as the number of restaurant inspections) and in terms of outcomes (such as the prevalence of food-borne illnesses). In a specific example of making the link between interventions and health outcomes, Los Angeles County pioneered a method of grading restaurants on their performance during inspections (a method since emulated by many other local public health agencies) and in recent years has demonstrated a correlation between restaurant grading and a decrease in food-borne infections (Simon et al., 2005).

Existing state accreditation programs and perhaps the emerging national accreditation program tend to focus heavily on standards for cross-cutting practices rather than standards related to implementation of specific, evidence-based public health programs, policies, and interventions (i.e., administrative processes versus programmatic content). Although that strategy has its strengths (such as ensuring that most or all public health agencies meet fundamental requirements and have basic tools and capacities), there is little or no research to show how such generic practices, usually acknowledged as useful or effective by practitioners, are related to implementation of evidence-based programs, policies, and interventions. (The committee notes that the public health accreditation process includes a measure of the use of evidence-based interventions.) A growing evidence base will be needed to inform public health leaders and practitioners as to which types of practices are effective in supporting successful implementation of efficacious and cost-effective programs, policies, or interventions.

Distributed Governance (and Accountabilities) in Complex Systems

To create a framework for holding other parties in the population health system accountable, other types of strategies are needed that serve a complex system in which multiple independent entities each hold a piece of the solution. Complexity theory would mandate a continually adapting governance process. The history and operating style of the public health agency mirrors in some ways those of public administrative structures and even of large organizations in the private sector. State and local public health agencies have traditionally been bureaucratic and operated in a linear, predictable, and planned manner and, with the exception of the executive-branch line of command, operated largely independently of any other entities.

For a variety of reasons, traditional modes of governance and action in public health need to be complemented with alternative approaches that depend on the specific problem at hand. That is due partly to the widespread recognition in public health that the government public health infrastructure generally "owns" neither the problems nor the solutions and thus needs to engage and collaborate with multiple stakeholders to find effective new ways to improve population health. The participation of multiple stakeholders creates the possibility of unpredictability and multiple mutually incompatible or incomprehensible terminologies, expertise, skill sets, and worldviews.

The literature on complexity theory and adaptive networks offers potential solutions, models, and road maps to help those who find themselves part of complex assemblages of government agencies, private-sector companies, nonprofit organizations, and various community groups. For example, Bovaird (2008) has written that expectations of system predictability must be modulated, and the typical process of strategic planning may need to give way to strategic management and "metaplanning" (for example, a more flexible set of approaches). Teisman (2008) has noted that self-organization may be a source of system evolution, and this would certainly apply to health systems in which no one is "in charge" and there are few or no common laws or statutes to structure governance. Flexible, adaptive systems can adjust to changing circumstances, such as new health data and emerging consequences of global climate change, and can develop strategies to keep on course (for example, sustaining previous gains and providing essential services) and to respond to new demands (Bovaird, 2008). In such systems, the public health agency does not have the authority to coordinate or align, but it could influence political leadership to create, with public-sector and private-sector partners, a policy context (statutes, financial incentives, and so on) to encourage alignment of interests. However, constantly changing and adapting systems will resist rigid governance structures, and other mechanisms will be needed (the committee will discuss these possibilities in a future report).

MEASUREMENT AND ACCOUNTABILITY IN THE FUTURE

As discussed in this chapter, there is a need to develop a model or framework for accountability for action on the broader determinants of health to improve population health. Although the full spectrum of system stakeholders have a role to play in accountability, the public health agencies form the core of the health system (defined as the joint capacities and activities of public health agencies, other government agencies, and multiple stakeholders outside government, including communities), and the federal government is an important funder of public health activities at the national, state, and local levels. That is why the committee believes that HHS is well positioned to act as a convener of all stakeholders in a process of broad-based planning and building on performance-measurement efforts already in existence in some parts of the health system or in other sectors.

The committee emphasizes that it is not calling for a federal mechanism for establishing or enforcing a national accountability system, but rather for federal public health agencies to convene and provide support to state and local agencies and their partners to develop a more detailed model and framework for accountability that may be used at all geographic levels. The committee also recognizes that the success of a health-in-all-policies approach resides outside the public health agency and that the approach can best be furthered at the behest of a supportive executive (mayor, governor, or president). The approach can also be successful if public health officials are strongly supportive of it *and* if their agencies' legislative mandate calls for such an approach (this will be discussed in the committee's report on the law).

In its recommendation below, the committee refers to a performance-measurement system that consists of standard approaches and metrics.

Recommendation 7
The committee recommends that the Department of Health and Human Services work with relevant federal, state, and local public-sector and private-sector partners and stakeholders to
1. Facilitate the development of a performance-measurement system that promotes accountability among governmental and private-sector organizations that have responsibilities for protecting and improving population health at local, state, and national levels. The system should include measures of the inputs contributed by those organizations (e.g., capabilities, resources, activities, and programs) and should allow tracking of impact on intermediate and population health outcomes.
2. Support the implementation of the performance measurement system by

a. Educating and securing the acceptance of the system by policy-makers and partners.
b. Establishing data-collection mechanisms needed to construct accountability measures at appropriate intervals at local, state, and national levels.
c. Encouraging early adoption of the system by key government and nongovernmental public health organizations and use of the system for performance reporting, quality improvement, planning, and policy development.
d. Assessing and developing the necessary health-system capacity (e.g., personnel, training, technical resources, and organizational structures) for broader adoption of the framework, including specific strategies for steps to address nonperformance by accountable agencies and organizations.

Strategies to address nonperformance by public health agencies referred to in the above recommendation could range from technical assistance, training, and mentorship to direct oversight and assumption of responsibilities, as well as from consolidation with other jurisdictions (or regionalization) to pooling of resources or sharing of specific resources and expertise to increase agency capacity and meet performance standards to ensure that each person in every jurisdiction has access to a full set of public health services.[6] Such strategies would be applied in a stepwise fashion that would build capacity locally and improve the health of the community.

With regard to holding public health agencies accountable, the committee believes that it is imperative that mechanisms for process and performance measurement not be linked with strategies that withhold funding from jurisdictions. Such actions could have serious unintended consequences for vulnerable populations and could potentially deepen disparities in health outcomes. Various incentives can be used to motivate agencies to change—for example, offering benefits to those who find ways to work together constructively. The current environment of severely constrained resources and preparation for an uncertain or unclear future (in light of an aging population, technologic advances, geopolitical and infectious-disease threats, and changes in the clinical care delivery system) could compel public health leaders to consider innovative and unconventional solutions to position their agencies to demonstrate effectiveness and efficiency; ensuring this will also require incentives that are outside the scope of the present report.

If the new framework for measurement to support accountability for

---

[6] For example, Michigan established district health departments, giving jurisdictions choice on consolidation (Bates et al., 2010).

population health is to function, the committee believes that a continuing focused effort in an existing organization (such as the PHAB, but with a broader mandate) or a new accountability organization may be needed to develop accountability measures and to track and report commitments by public health agencies and other stakeholders. To help federal agencies, public health funders, and communities, the accountability organization would involve them in the development of accountability measures and reporting requirements. The accountability organization would need the capacity to understand the underlying logic model that links the actions taken by public health agencies and stakeholders with intermediate and health outcomes so that it can help to identify the critical processes, resources, and capabilities of each stakeholder that are central to the intervention strategy. Such an organization

- Could assist in the measurement and reporting of performance of nongovernment public health stakeholders that are accountable for upholding mutual accountability "compacts" formed with others in improving community health outcomes.
- Could validate and serve as a repository of accountability indicators and serve as a facilitator of process integrity and objectivity on behalf of funders, taxpayers, and communities.
- Would need to be constituted appropriately to incorporate necessary expertise and demonstrate needed independence.

TYPES AND EXAMPLES OF NEEDED
ACCOUNTABILITY MEASURES

There are various ways to measure accountability of stakeholders in the health system. For clinical care services delivered in public health department clinics, it may be most reasonable to consider measurement strategies that are used in the clinical care delivery sector. Such strategies (Healthcare Effectiveness Data and Information Set [HEDIS] measures for instance) are likely to grow in importance in the wake of major changes to the clinical care delivery system, and the clinical services provided in public health may also change as a result of a decrease, due to the ACA, in the number of uninsured people who need the immunization, family-planning, or communicable-disease services offered by clinics that public health agencies operate.

With regard to funding of public health agencies, a local system of public health accounts is needed to enable management to understand how well resources are aligned with interventions and outcomes. As noted in Chapter 1, measurement of financial resources and their effects on services and outcomes is inadequate. Public health agencies do not collect data in a standardized way to link decisions on how resources are spent at the local level (in the health department) with the population health outcomes that they are designed to improve. And, as discussed in this chapter and elsewhere in this report, the linking of inputs and outcomes is not a simple or straightforward process, for a variety of reasons (see Box 4-4 for a discussion of so-called scorecards). Information is needed not merely by funding stream or categorical program; rather it is needed as a type of accounting— what resources go toward what health outcomes, and what is the effect? The committee began to discuss this topic and expects to gather additional information in preparing its third report.

For many stakeholders in the health system, developing accountability measures has been challenging for several reasons. Many in the business sector or non-health-related parts of the nonprofit sector have not always seen themselves as stakeholders in health. There may be data gaps or difficulties in gathering needed data, and evidence available to guide the selection of measures may be sparse. Such measurement systems as HEDIS may serve as a partial model, but there are considerable differences, compared with clinical settings (described in more detail earlier in this chapter), in the ability to link cause and effect in population health and in how accountability is traced both in the government public health infrastructure (which is supported by taxpayers and accountable to them and to elected officials) and among the many stakeholders in the system (where accountabilities are much less clearly defined and certainly more difficult to monitor and evaluate). However, the committee believes that the concerted efforts of national public health leaders, with support from public health systems and services research and input from communities, can move the field toward developing and implementing good performance measures that can be adopted by implementers and those holding them accountable. Criteria for selecting such measures may include face validity (meaningfulness, relevance, and understandability), feasibility (availability or collectability of data), methodologic soundness (validity and reliability), and fairness (to the stakeholders whose performance they will evaluate).

The set of performance measures used may differ, depending on a community's identified needs and priorities, on the mix of stakeholders, and on the expectations of funders. The Ten Essential Public Health Services (see Box 4-2) may also serve as a tool for identifying measures to assess. See Table 4-1 for some examples of possible measures of performance for agreed-on strategies.

Over the last few decades, efforts to measure and report quality and performance related to health have increased. Spurred by such employer initiatives as the Leapfrog programs for reporting hospital-service quality, such government initiatives as Medicare quality measures for ambulatory care and hospitals, and health care quality organization standards of the

BOX 4-4
Improving the Next Generation of "Scorecards"

Several sets of indicators have been developed or have been made available to the public in the last 2 decades. Prominent examples include the State of the USA (SUSA) health measures (developed as part of a national, federally driven key-indicators effort), the Community Health Status Indicators effort (supported by HHS agencies and several nonprofit organizations), and the County Health Rankings (developed by academic researchers with foundation support) (Community Health Status Indicators, 2009; County Health Rankings, 2009; SUSA, 2010).

Some indicator sets are sometimes called scorecards, and the committee believes that it is important to address this terminology. Although these indicator sets (discussed in Chapter 2) attempt to provide snapshots of health by county or by state (in the case of SUSA) and can speak volumes about the needs and challenges in a given community, the snapshots generally are not intended to and do not inform about the performance of the public health agencies in the communities and about the resources available to them. These sets also provide only limited information about the underlying determinants of health (most commonly, data on educational attainment and income). It is the committee's understanding that true scorecards (which are available in many fields, including health) are intended to convey information about performance (such as the quality of services provided) either for internal quality-improvement purposes or for external communication, but some of the indicator sets currently called scorecards are in fact unable to provide the type of information a true scorecard would give. The committee believes that policy-makers and the public cannot draw useful inferences about public health agency competence or capabilities from these so-called scorecards (in their most common current formats). Examples of true scorecards may be found in the clinical

National Committee on Quality Assurance, the National Quality Forum (NQF), and others, the medical care delivery system has begun to report performance and quality-improvement activities linking process to health outcomes. What the present committee recommends should not be considered in isolation from the efforts of those groups, and existing efforts should be incorporated when possible and when they are pertinent to population health. For example, the Centers for Disease Control and Prevention National Public Health Performance Standards program is designed to measure public health practices at the state and local levels and provides the tool Mobilizing for Action through Planning and Partnerships, which evaluates the capacity of local public health systems to conduct the Ten Essential Public Health Services. In the clinical care setting, the NQF uses continuous quality improvement as part of its vision, which is a facet of a measurement framework for accountability recommended by the committee. The national context, but, as discussed in this chapter and elsewhere in this report, the clinical frameworks do not translate easily to public health practice.

The committee believes that it is crucial that future indicator sets described as community scorecards look not only at important distal health outcomes and determinants (largely the measures of community health discussed in Chapters 2 and 3) but also at their interrelationships with upstream underlying processes and policies, which may differ at the local, state, and national levels. Given that health outcomes are the products of a chain of proximal and distal influences, the interrelationships among health and its determinants should serve as an organizing framework for future measurement of health outcomes. Rather than presenting a "flat-file" list of health indicators, for every distal health outcome of importance, future efforts would map out the causal web of determinants that affect outcomes and the sequence of upstream activities that enable communities to alter the determinants. The systems-modeling activities described and called for in Chapter 3 could transform this kind of performance measurement by leading to a next generation of health indicators that measure performance along complex and nonlinear causal pathways and at the national, state, and local levels. It would require research and development to identify the most important health outcomes at the distal end of the pathway, the activities that are effective at each stage of influence, and the best metrics for each indicator. To accomplish that, changes in survey administration and data collection and analysis will be necessary. As discussed in Chapter 3, there may be value in individual health data from electronic health records that could be collectively analyzed with appropriate privacy and security safeguards (such as aggregation) to complement the understanding of community or population health. Without such understanding, the implementation of policies and other strategies that affect social, environmental, and behavioral determinants cannot be measured, monitored, and improved.

accreditation effort, as discussed earlier, will also be a useful tool as it moves forward in its development.

Implementation of the Measurement Framework for Accountability

Chapter 1 discusses the causes, and causes of causes, that lead to the untoward health outcomes of infant mortality and cardiovascular disease. As is true for the vast majority of conditions or illnesses, neither of those outcomes is amenable to improvements that are influenced solely by public health agencies. A variety of stakeholders are necessary to alter the micro and macro societal conditions in which infants die and people suffer heart attacks and congestive heart failure. Beyond the most macro level—the deeply embedded socioeconomic realities that characterize the nation—employers, community organizations, clinical care providers, schools, busi-

TABLE 4-1 Examples of Measures of Common Agreed-on Strategies

Sample Measure	Stakeholder
Number of employers who have voluntarily adopted and complied with smoke-free workplace policies	Business, nonprofits
Number of (nonchain) restaurants voluntarily posting or complying with requirements for disclosure of nutritional information	Business (retail)
School adherence to nutrition guidelines, including removal of some vending-machine products	Schools
Planning and zoning decisions consistent with local needs	Planning department
Small-business compliance with smoking bans (something intermediate to) high school graduation rates	Business Schools, community-services agencies
Percentage of community housing that is affordable (give parameters)	Planning department, local government, developers
Percentage of community housing that is safe and livable (give parameters)	Police, planning, local government, community groups, faith-based organizations
Percentage of poor children (specify percentage of federal poverty level) who receive early-childhood interventions (from public health and other social-service agencies)	Public health agency, social services, nonprofit organizations, including advocacy groups and philanthropic organizations
Percentage of medical-insurance plans that implement health-literacy education; percentage of medical-insurance plans or medical care providers that adopt health-literacy strategies and implement steps to increase cultural competence of their staff; measures of health literacy in adolescents	Clinical care Schools
Percentage of employers that provide wellness services to employees	Business, employers
Percentage of employers who adopt policies supportive of breastfeeding mothers (including dedicated, acceptable space and time to pump)	Business, employers
Percentage of baby-friendly (that is, breastfeeding-supportive) hospitals (specific parameters have been described elsewhere)	Clinical care

nesses, and many others can undertake strategies that address one or both of those outcomes (and many others).

For example, in a community that has unacceptable infant mortality, the local public health agency might serve as the convener of stakeholders, alerting other community organizations to the problem's root causes by presenting evidence of associations between different types of changeable risk factors and infant outcomes. In doing so, it might identify weaknesses in the local programs, services, and interventions available to prevent unplanned pregnancies and poor birth outcomes. Those convened might also engage a broader circle of participants who are in a position to influence environmental changes. Those convened could then consider, plan, and deploy an array of strategies. After reaching consensus on the top (most effective, evidence-based, and locally appropriate) strategies to be undertaken, the coalition could develop agreements with various stakeholders who would all commit to playing a concrete role in improving the outcome of concern. For example, the local public health or social services agencies would commit to better links to clinical care providers who are working with newly pregnant women to ensure that at-risk women receive case management and other essential services. The public health agency and clinical care providers in the community might develop agreements to ensure that no pregnant woman misses prenatal care services because of insurance status or difficulty in accessing a provider. Local businesses that cater to women and families could join in a mass-media and social marketing campaign on the importance of prenatal care. Schools could initiate or intensify efforts to educate adolescents about family planning and refer them to clinical services (as part of a broader effort to delay sexual activity and improve awareness and behaviors).

A broader coalition might work to alter the community environment more substantially. For example, local employers and businesses learning of the relationship of secondhand smoke to poor infant outcomes might commit to initiating or enhancing smoke-free environments to diminish exposure of pregnant women and alter the behaviors of other members of the community. Schools boards, learning of the relationship between graduation rates and infant mortality, might be persuaded to redouble efforts to increase graduation. Town planners, alerted to an association between early sexual activity and lack of recreational outlets, might agree to work to design programs and build facilities to serve adolescents. Food retailers, made more aware of the relationship between nutrition and birth outcomes, might commit to developing food and menu labeling as part of a communication effort. The process of involving those many organizations could include developing a coalition that could acquire formal nonprofit status (501(c)3) and apply for funding from relevant private and public-sector funders.

Implementing a measurement framework for accountability could include agreements and contracts (in cases in which funding is provided) and a variety of tools for communicating with the public on the status and progress of the community's joint efforts (for example, through newsletters, news releases, and monthly, quarterly, or annual reports). Evidence-based indicators could be selected to help the community to hold accountable all stakeholders who have agreed to contribute to the initiative in some manner. Indicators could include an array of process measures, such as the percentage of newly pregnant women receiving social support (the Women, Infants, and Children federal food and nutrition program and food stamps) who are referred for additional services, a measure of the level of tracking and follow-up of women who do not access needed services, indicators of clinicians' attempts to initiate smoking cessation in pregnant women, measures of mass-media and other communication outputs, and the percentage of businesses that adopt smoke-free policies to decrease exposure of pregnant women. As the work progresses, indicators that can be used to hold stakeholders accountable will become more refined, interventions will also be fine-tuned, efforts to collect data will begin to produce results, and the public will have regularly updated information about progress in addressing one of the community's top health needs.

The committee believes that the task of identifying performance measures can be simplified under the proposed framework because, for the most part, performance measures need to be measures of execution of strategies or of immediate outcomes of execution.

CONCLUDING OBSERVATIONS

In this chapter, the committee has outlined the three components of a measurement system for accountability that can be applied to the entire health system, from public health agencies to a vast array of stakeholders, and made a recommendation describing standard approaches and measures for implementing the framework in the context of both contract accountability and mutual or compact accountability.

Accountability requires measurements that track resources to outcomes; in general, these measures are not yet developed. Accountability is primarily for processes required by funders or agreed to by those in mutual accountability arrangements—processes over which organizations have control, rather than health outcomes for which public health is often only one of many contributors and determinants and therefore cannot be held directly accountable.

Simple measures of accountability (clear lines from inputs to outputs) based on quantified improvements in health outcomes, although desirable, are not possible, so the three-part, more complex framework of accountability measurement and continuous quality improvement presented in the report is needed. This measurement strategy can be operationalized across the spectrum of degree of certainty about best practices and so avoids "accountability paralysis" from lack of precise science. The strategy can be operationalized in both contract and compact operating environments and for all stakeholders, and the principles embodied are applicable at national, state, and local levels. Priority steps to develop and implement the measurement framework should be taken.

REFERENCES

Alameda County Public Health Department. 2008. *Life and Death from Unnatural Causes: Health and Social Inequity in Alameda County.* Oakland, CA: Alameda County Public Health Department.

Baicker, K., D. Cutler, and Z. Song. 2010. Workplace wellness programs can generate savings. *Health Affairs* 29(2):304-311.

Bates, L. J., B. A. Lafrancois, and R. E. Santerre. 2010. An empirical study of the consolidation of local public health services in connecticut. *Public Choice* DOI 10.1007/s11127-010-9606-9.

Benjamin, G., M. Fallon, P. E. Jarris, and P. Libbey. 2006 (September). *Final Recommendations for a Voluntary National Accreditation Program for State and Local Public Health Departments.* Alexandria, VA: PHAB.

Berwick, D. M. 2002. A user's manual for the IOM's 'quality chasm' report. *Health Affairs* 21(3):80-90.

Bourgeois, F., W. W. Simmons, K. Olson, J. S. Brownstein, and K. D. Mandi. 2008. Evaluation of influenza prevention in the workplace using a personally controlled health record: Randomized controlled trial. *Journal of Medical Internet Research* 10(1):e5.

Bovaird, T. 2008. Emergent strategic management and planning mechanisms in complex adaptive systems: The case of the UK best value initiative. *Public Management Review* 10(3):319-340.

CDC (Centers for Disease Control and Prevention). 2010. *Health Impact Assessment: Fact Sheet.* Atlanta, GA: CDC.

Communities Count. 2008. Summary of Social and Health Indicators: Communities Count 2008: Executive summary. In *Communities Count 2008: Social and health indicators across King County.* Seattle, WA: Communities County. Pp. iv-xi.

Community Health Status Indicators. 2009. *About the Community Health Status Indicators Project.* http://www.communityhealth.hhs.gov/AboutTheProject.aspx?GeogCD=&PeerStrat=&state=&county= (January 6, 2010).

County Health Rankings. 2009. *About the Community Health Status Indicators Project.* http://www.countyhealthrankings.org/latest-news/how-washington-county-residents-stay-healthy (January 6, 2010).

Department of Population Health Sciences. 2008. *Wisconsin County Health Rankings—2008.* Madison: University of Wisconsin School of Medicine and Public Health.

EPA (Environmental Protection Agency). 2010. *HUD-DOT-EPA Interagency Partnership for Sustainable Communities.* http://www.epa.gov/smartgrowth/partnership/index.html (September 8, 2010).

Franco, M., A.V. Diez-Roux, J. A. Nettleton, M. Lazo, F. Brancati, B. Caballero, T. Glass, and L. V. Moore. 2009. Availability of healthy foods and dietary patterns: The multi-ethnic study of atherosclerosis. *American Journal of Clinical Nutrition* 89(3):897-904.

Glasgow, R. E. 2010. HMC research translation: Speculations about making it real and going to scale. *American Journal of Health Behavior* 34(6):833-840.

Goetzel, R. Z., and R. J. Ozminkowski. 2008. The health and cost benefits of work site health-promotion programs. *Annual Review of Public Health* 29:303-323.

Guide to Community Preventive Services. 2010. *What Is the Community Guide?* http://www.thecommunityguide.org/index.html (August 16, 2010).

The Healthy Development Measurement Tool. 2006. *Case Studies: Hope SF-Redevelopment of San Francisco's Public Housing.* http://www.thehdmt.org/case_studies.php (September 5, 2010).

Heinen, L., and H. Darling. 2009. Addressing obesity in the workplace: The role of employers. *Milbank Quarterly* 87(1):101-122.

HHS (Department of Health and Human Services). 2010. *Affordable Care Act: Laying the Foundation for Prevention.* http://www.healthreform.gov/about/index.html (June 22, 2010).

HHS and CDC. 2008. *Local Public Health Governance Performance Assessment: Model Standards.* Washington, DC: HHS and CDC.

Houle, B., and M. Siegel. 2009. Smoker-free workplace policies: Developing a model of public health consequences of workplace policies barring employment to smokers. *Tobacco Control* 18(1):64-69.

IOM (Institute of Medicine). 1988. *The Future of Public Health.* Washington, DC: National Academy Press.

IOM. 1997. *Improving Health in the Community: A Role for Performance Monitoring.* Washington, DC: National Academy Press.

IOM. 2001. *Crossing the Quality Chasm: A New Health System for the 21st Century.* Washington, DC: National Academy Press.

IOM. 2003a. *The Future of the Public's Health in the 21st Century.* Washington, DC: The National Academies Press.

IOM. 2003b. The Governmental Public Health Infrastructure. In *The Future of the Public's Health.* Washington, DC: The National Academies Press. Pp. 96-177.

Keall, M., M. G. Baker, P. Howden-Chapman, M. Cunning, and D. Ormandy. 2010. Assessing housing quality and its impact on health, safety and sustainability. *Journal of Epidemiology and Community Health* 64(9):765-71.

Koivusalo, M. 2010. The state of health in all policies (HiAP) in the European Union: Potential and pitfalls. *Journal of Epidemiology and Community Health* 64:500-503.

Krieger, J., and D. L. Higgins. 2002. Housing and health: Time again for public health action. *American Journal of Public Health* 92(5):758-768.

Lemstra, M., and C. Neudorf. 2008. *Health Disparity in Saskatoon: Analysis to Intervention.* http://www.uphn.ca/doc/public/HealthDisaparitiesinSaskatoonExecutiveSummary.pdf (January 2010).

MacDonald, J. M., R. J. Strokes, D.A. Cohen, A. Kofner, and G. K. Ridgeway. 2010 The effect of light rail transit on body mass index and physical activity. *American Journal of Preventive Medicine* 39(2):105-112.

Michigan Department of Community Health. 2008a. *Increasing Access to Healthy Foods: Michigan's New Property Tax Incentive for Retail Food Establishments (Public Act 231 of 2008).* Lansing: Michigan Department of Community Health.

Michigan Department of Community Health. 2008b. *Reducing infant mortality in Michigan: Lessons from the field.* Lansing: Michigan Department of Community Health.

NACCHO (National Association of County and City Health Officials). 2009a. Integrating performance improvement processes: MAPP, National Public Health Performance Standards, and accreditation. Washington, DC: NACCHO.

NACCHO. 2009b. Mobilizing for Action through Planning and Partnerships and the National Public Health Performance Standards Program: What is the relationship? Washington, DC: NACCHO.

National Center for Appropriate Technology. 2010. *Smart growth resource: HUD, DOT and EPA announce interagency partnership for sustainable communities.* http://www.smartgrowth.org/misc/default.asp?art=83&res=1024 (September 2, 2010).

NPLAN (National Policy and Legal Analysis Network). 2009. *Model Menue Labeling Ordinance.* Oakland, CA: National Policy and Legal Analysis Network.

NYC (New York City) Department of City Planning. 2010. *Fresh Food Stores: Overview.* http://home2.nyc.gov/html/dcp/html/fresh/index.shtml (September 20, 2010).

OECD (Organisation for European Economic Co-operation). 2009. *Mututal Accountablity.* Paris, France: OECD.

Office of Health Assessment and Epidemiology. 2010. *Life Expectancy in Los Angeles County: How Long Do We Live and Why? A Cities and Communities Health Report.* Los Angeles, CA: County of Los Angeles Department of Public Health.

Okie, S. 2007. The employer as health coach. *New England Journal of Medicine* 357(15): 1465-1469.

Ozminkowski, R. J., D. Ling, R. Z. Goetzel, J. A. Bruno, K. R. Rutter, F. Isaac, and S. Wang. 2002. Long-term impact of Johnson & Johnson's Health & Wellness Program on health care utilization and expenditures. *Journal of Occupational and Environmental Medicine* 44(1):21-29.

PHAB (Public Health Accreditation Board). 2009. Proposed state standards and measures, adopted by the PHAB board of directors, July 16, 2009 for PHAB Beta Test. Alexandria, VA: PHAB.

PHAB. 2010. *E-Newsletter: Public Health Accreditation Board.* http://archive.constantcontact. com/fs030/1102084465533/archive/1103695445388.html (September 8, 2010).

Public Health Functions Steering Committee. 1994. *The Public Health Workforce: An Agenda for the 21st Century. Full Report of the Public Health Functions Project.* Washington, DC: HHS.

RWJF (Robert Wood Johnson Foundation) and W.K. Kellogg Foundation. 2006. *Turning Point Performance Management Collaborative.* http://www.turningpointprogram.org/ (September 2, 2010).

Seattle and King County Public Health Department. 2010. *King County Community Health Indicators.* http://www.kingcounty.gov/healthservices/health/data/chi.aspx (January 6, 2010).

Simon, P. A., P. Leslie, G. Run, G. Z. Jin, R. Reporter, A. Aguirre, and J. E. Fielding. 2005. Impact of restaurant hygiene grade cards on foodborne-disease hospitalizations in Los Angeles County. *Journal of Environmental Health* 46(7):32-36.

Simon, P., C. J. Jarosz, T. Kuo, and J. E. Fielding. 2008. *Menu Labeling as a Potential Strategy for Combating the Obesity Epidemic: A Health Impact Assessment (HIA).* Los Angeles, CA: Los Angeles County Department of Public Health.

Summers, C., L. Cohen, A. Havusha, F. Sliger, and T. Farley. 2009. *Take Care New York 2012: A Policy for a Healthier New York City.* New York, NY: New York City Department of Health and Mental Hygiene.

SUSA (State of the USA). 2010. *The State of the USA.* http://www.stateoftheusa.org (September 1, 2010).

Syme, S. L., and M. L. Ritterman. 2009. The importance of community development for health and well-being. *Community Development Investment Review* 5(3):1-13.

Teisman, G. 2008. Complexity and management of improvement programmes: An evolutionary approach. *Public Management Review* 10(3):341-359.

University of Wisconsin Population Health Institute. 2010. *Mobilizing Action Toward Community Health (MATCH): Population health metrics, solid partnerships, and real incentives.* http://uwphi.pophealth.wisc.edu/pha/match.htm (June 10, 2010).

USDA (United States Department of Agriculture). 2010. *About the Food Environment Atlas.* http://ers.usda.gov/FoodAtlas/about.htm (September 8, 2010).

White House Task Force on Childhood Obesity. 2010. *Solving the Problem of Childhood Obesity Within a Generation.* Washington, DC: Executive Office of the President of the United States.

World Bank. 2008. *Mutual Accountability.* New York, NY: United Nations Development Group.

Appendix A

Acronyms

ACA	Affordable Care Act, 2010
AHR	America's Health Rankings
AHRQ	Agency for Healthcare Research and Quality
ASTHO	Association of State and Territorial Health Officials
BMI	body mass index
BRFSS	Behavioral Risk Factor Surveillance System
CDC	Centers for Disease Control and Prevention
CHCF	California HealthCare Foundation
CHDI	Community Health Data Initiative
CHIS	California Health Interview Survey
CHR	county health rankings
CHSI	Community Health Status Indicators
CMS	Centers for Medicare and Medicaid Services
CVD	cardiovascular disease
DALY	disability-adjusted life year
DHEW	Department of Health, Education, and Welfare
DOT	Department of Transportation
EHR	electronic health record
EPA	Environmental Protection Agency

GAO	Government Accountability Office
GDP	gross domestic product
HALE	health-adjusted life expectancy
HALY	health-adjusted life year
HHS	Department of Health and Human Services
HIA	health impact assessment
HP 2010	Healthy People 2010
HRQL	health-related quality of life
HUD	Department of Housing and Urban Development
IOM	Institute of Medicine
MATCH	Mobilizing Action Toward Community Health
NACCHO	National Association of County and City Health Officials
NAS	National Academy of Sciences
NCHS	National Center for Health Statistics
NCQA	National Committee for Quality Assurance
NCVHS	National Committee on Vital and Health Statistics
NHANES	National Health and Nutrition Examination Survey
NHIS	National Health Interview Survey
NICE	National Institute for Health and Clinical Excellence
NIH	National Institutes of Health
NPHPPHC	National Prevention, Health Promotion, and Public Health Council
NQF	National Quality Form
OECD	Organisation for Economic Co-operation and Development
PHAB	Public Health Acceditation Board
QALY	quality-adjusted life year
SUSA	State of the USA
TFAH	Trust for America's Health

Appendix B

National and Community
Health Data Sets

NATIONAL DATA SETS

The most readily available health-outcomes data for the United States are mortality data, which are derived from death certificates and population health surveys and contain self-reported health and functional status. The national surveys most often used are the Behavioral Risk Factors Surveillance System (BRFSS) and the National Health Interview Survey (NHIS), which provide data annually, and the National Health and Nutrition Examination Survey (NHANES), which provides data every 2 years (CDC, 2008, 2009a, 2009b).

The Behavioral Risk Factors Surveillance System

BRFSS is a cross-sectional telephone-based survey that collects information on changes in health conditions and risk factors (Mokdad, 2009). State health departments conduct BRFSS with support and design from the Centers for Disease Control and Prevention (CDC). Most states use BRFSS as their primary source of chronic-disease data for evaluating health behaviors in the population. BRFSS is the world's largest telephone survey and has 413,000 adult participants each year (Balluz, 2010); it is offered in English and Spanish (CDC, 2008). The goals of BRFSS are to assess public health status, define public health priorities, evaluate programs, stimulate research, and monitor trends (Balluz, 2010). BRFSS provides state-level estimates and estimates for selected metropolitan statistical areas that have 500 or more respondents. It collects demographic variables on race, sex, age, income categories, education level, and number of children in the household

(Mokdad, 2009). The BRFSS questionnaire is organized by core and optional modules and includes individual-level risk factors associated with causes of premature death (Mokdad, 2009). More detailed information on chronic conditions—including diabetes, cardiovascular health, high blood pressure, and adult asthma—are included in optional modules (Balluz, 2010).

The National Health Information Survey

NHIS, supported by the CDC's National Center for Health Statistics (NCHS), is a large-scale cross-sectional household interview survey. The survey includes information on population disease prevalence, extent of disability, and use of health care services and is offered in English, Spanish, and other languages. NHIS describes disease prevalence from self-reports of diagnoses received from clinicians (Burrows et al., 2007). The expected NHIS sample includes about 35,000–40,000 households with 75,000–100,000 persons of all ages. To provide state or local estimates of health outcomes and determinants of health, a few states and local areas, such as Wisconsin and New York City, conduct their own surveys based on the NHIS (and NHANES) method (CDC, 2009a; Parrish, 2010).

The National Health and Nutrition Examination Survey

NHANES is a "program of studies designed to assess the health and nutritional status of adults and children in the United States." It combines interviews with physical examinations and is conducted by NCHS (CDC, 2009a). A nationally representative sample of about 5,000 people are interviewed each year. NHANES includes demographic, socioeconomic, dietary, and health-related questions offered in English and Spanish. The examination component consists of medical, dental, and physiologic measurements, including laboratory tests. The data from the survey are used to determine the prevalence of major diseases and risk factors for diseases (CDC, 2009a).

Limitations of the Behavioral Risk Factors Surveillance System, the National Health Information Survey, and the National Health and Nutrition Examination Survey

BRFSS, NHIS, and NHANES all have limitations and challenges. BRFSS has a declining and low response rate (for example, 18 percent in California and a national median of 34 percent—a lower response rate than NHIS and NHANES) and inadequate time available for questions, responses are self-reported, data are available only at the state level (and some large jurisdictions), and the survey contains no biometric measurements. BRFSS includes few or no measures of newer constructs of community health, such as social cohesion, resilience, and literacy.

Data in national data sets can sometimes be stratified for a state, or state data may be available from a state's own efforts (for example, a state-based *Health and Nutrition Examination Survey*), but local leaders who seek statistics for their county, city, or census tract face challenges in obtaining geocodable data. The obstacles are sometimes methodologic—as when sample sizes or survey techniques are problematic in sparsely populated rural communities—but often the difficulty is that source agencies have done little either to collect the data or, when the data are available, to make the information readily available to the typical decision-maker.

Procedures used by researchers to extract geocodable microdata from agency data warehouses or to file paperwork for agency approvals to integrate such data often pose a formidable barrier for busy policy-makers or staff of public health agencies. Making such data accessible to those important users requires efforts at a high level to develop a front end that enables users to obtain available statistics easily and to cross government agency silos (such as planning, zoning, transportation, and education) to gather and report relevant local data from multiple sources in a useful way.

NHIS does provide health status information on a representative sample of Americans, but it does not provide state or local estimates. BRFSS provides state estimates, but it does not provide local data, and it provides minimal data on children. To complement what they obtain from BRFSS, 16 states provide funding to enhance their BRFSS samples with substate sampling strata to generate their own representative local data sets, and others add their own modules on other topics of interest to them. Eleven states have established separate comprehensive surveys independent of BRFSS, such as the California Health Interview Survey (CHIS), to meet their needs for local and state data not being served by BRFSS (UCLA Center for Health Policy Research, 2008), and 10 states conduct independent surveys to assess the health of children (UCLA Center for Healthier Children, 2010).

Several states conduct city or county surveys on the basis of BRFSS and have been able to use the data to monitor trends and risks (CDC, 2009b), but overall the data are not adequate for use at the local level (and cannot measure inequalities in health that occur at the community level and among population subgroups), because samples are too small for calculating reliable estimates (Parrish, 2010). NHIS and NHANES provide only national and some large regional estimates because of their sampling schemes and relatively small samples. Because a premium is placed on statistical rigor and because securing financing for the surveys and supplements is complex, these sources do not adapt rapidly to and maximize opportunities afforded by available communication technologies. In addition, data are not available as rapidly as needed, and some content reflects the needs of funders rather than the overall needs of public health.

COMMUNITY DATA SETS

One early effort in population health measurement and reporting is America's Health Rankings (AHR), which was begun in 1990 and provides a scorecard of health determinants and health-outcome measures and an overall ranking for each state (America's Health Rankings, 2009). In 2009, a county analogue to AHR, the County Health Rankings, was released; it ranks counties in each state on specific health measures (County Health Rankings, 2010a). The Community Health Status Indicators (CHSI) activity was initiated in 2000 and relaunched in 2006 by a collaborative group of federal, state, and local public health representation and nonprofit and academic partners (County Health Rankings, 2009).[1] CHSI provides detailed health (and related) measures by county and allows users to compare peer counties (for example, counties with similar sociodemographic characteristics).

The interest in and proliferation of health indicators is linked to a national concern about health-related costs and health-system effectiveness and to a federal initiative on key national indicators (for example, related to population, economy, environment, health, education, and commerce) that began early in the 21st century. In 2003, the General Accounting Office (GAO), now the Government Accountability Office, held a forum on key national indicators in collaboration with the National Academies (GAO, 2003). In 2003 and 2004, GAO prepared several reports on the key indicators initiative; in 2004, the Organisation for Economic Co-operation and Development reported on this subject in its World Forum on Key Indicators (GAO, 2004). The Academies continue to serve as the secretariat for the effort, supporting several activities that include a recent Institute of Medicine committee convened to identify 20 health indicators in three domains (health outcomes, health-related behaviors, and medical care delivery systems) to track progress in health and health care (IOM, 2009). These will be incorporated into the State of the USA (SUSA) project, which is likely to be the repository for the Key National Indicators required by the Affordable Care Act in subjects including health and managed by the

---

[1] Partners include the Centers for Disease Control and Prevention, the National Institutes of Health National Library of Medicine, the Health Resources Services Administration, the Public Health Foundation, the Association of State and Territorial Health Officials, the National Association of County and City Health Officials, the National Association of Local Boards of Health, and the Johns Hopkins University School of Public Health (County Health Rankings, 2010b).

National Academies (more information is available on the SUSA website[2]; see Public Law 111-148).

Tables B-1 (national indicator sets) and B-2 (community indicator sets) present samples of the numerous indicator sets in existence. Those represented in the table were chosen because they are the best known and are representative sets regarding the types of indications used currently in the United States. To view more exhaustive reviews of the existing data sets, see Public Health Institute (2010) and Wold (2008).

REFERENCES

Alameda County Public Health Department. 2008. *Life and Death from Unnatural Causes: Health and Social Inequity in Alameda County.* Oakland, CA: Alameda County Public Health Department.

America's Health Rankings. 2009. *A Call to Action for Individuals and Their Communities.* Minnetonka, MN: United Health Foundation.

America's Health Rankings. 2010. *Definitions of Components: Core Measures and Supplemental Measures.* http://www.americashealthrankings.org/2009/component.aspx (June 4, 2010).

Balluz, L. 2010. (January 21, 2010). *Behavioral Risk Factor Surveillance System (BRFSS).* Presentation to the IOM Committee on Public Health Strategies to Improve Health. Washington, DC: IOM.

Burrows, N. R., S. Parekh, Y. Li, L. S. Geiss, and CDC. 2007. Prevalence of self-reported cardiovascular disease among persons aged >35 years with diabetes—United States, 1997–2005. *Morbidity and Mortality Weekly Report* 56(43):1129-1132.

CDC (Centers for Disease Control and Prevention). 2008. *Behavioral Risk Factor Surveillance System: About the BRFSS.* http://www.cdc.gov/brfss/about.htm (January 1, 2010).

CDC. 2009a. *About the National Health Interview Survey.* http://www.cdc.gov/nchs/nhis/about_nhis.htm (January 6, 2010).

CDC. 2009b. *Overview: BRFSS 2008.* http://www.cdc.gov/brfss/technical_infodata/survey-data/2008/overview_08.rtf (January 6, 2010).

Community Health Status Indicators. 2009. *Community Health Status Indicators Project Fact Sheet.* Washington, DC: HHS.

Community Health Status Indicators Project Working Group. 2009. *Data Sources, Definitions, and Notes for CHSI 2009.* Washington, DC.: Department of Health and Human Services.

County Health Rankings. 2009. *About the Community Health Status Indicators Project.* http://www.countyhealthrankings.org/latest-news/how-washington-county-residents-stay-healthy (January 6, 2010).

County Health Rankings. 2010a. *Data Collection Process.* http://www.countyhealthrankings.org/about-project/data-collection-process (February 17, 2010).

County Health Rankings. 2010b. *How Healthy Is Your County? New County Health Rankings Give First County-by-county Snapshot of Health in Each State.* http://www.countyhealthrankings.org/latest-news/healthday-county-county-report-sizes-americans-health (February 17, 2010).

GAO (Government Accountability Office). 2003. *Forum on Key National Indicators.* Washington, DC: GAO.

---

[2] See http://www.stateoftheusa.org/.

GAO. 2004. *Informing Our Nation: Improving How to Understand and Assess the USA's Position and Progress*. Washington, DC: GAO.

HHS (Department of Health and Human Services). 2009a. *Healthy People 2020 Framework*. http://www.healthypeople.gov/hp2020/objectives/framework.aspx (April 28, 2010).

HHS. 2009b. *Healthy People 2020 Public Meetings—2009 Draft Objectives*. Washington, DC: Department of Health and Human Services.

IOM (Institute of Medicine). 2009. *State of the USA Health Indicators: Letter Report*. Washington, DC: The National Academies Press.

Mokdad, A. H. 2009. The Behavioral Risk Factors Surveillance System: Past, present, and future. *Annual Review of Public Health* 30:43-54.

Parrish, R. G. 2010. Measuring population health outcomes. *Preventing Chronic Disease Public Health Research, Practice and Policy* 7(4). http://www.cdc.gov/pcd/issues/2010/jul/10_0005.htm. (July 4, 2010).

Public Health Institute. 2010. *Data Sets, Data Platforms, Data Utility: Resource Compendium*. Oakland, CA: Public Health Institute.

Saskatoon Regional Health Authority. 2007. *2006-2007 Annual Report to the Minister of Health and the Minister of Healthy Living Services*. Saskatoon, Canada: Saskatoon Regional Health Authority.

Seattle and King County Public Health. 2010. *King County Community Health Indicators*. http://www.kingcounty.gov/healthservices/health/data/chi.aspx (January 6, 2010).

Summers, C., L. Cohen, A. Havusha, F. Sliger, and T. Farley. 2009. *Take Care New York 2012: A Policy for a Healthier New York City*. New York: New York City Department of Health and Mental Hygiene.

SUSA (State of the USA). 2010a. *Mission*. http://www.stateoftheusa.org/about/mission (June 11, 2010).

SUSA. 2010b. *The State of the USA*. http://www.stateoftheusa.org (September 1, 2010).

Trust for America's Health. 2010. *State Data*. http://healthyamericans.org/states (October 15, 2010).

UCLA (University of California, Los Angeles) Center for Health Policy Research. 2008. *About CHIS*. http://www.askchis.com/about.html (September 1, 2010).

UCLA Center for Healthier Children. 2010. *Framework for System Transformation*. http://healthychild.ucla.edu/Transformation.asp (June 16, 2010).

Wold, C. 2008. *Health Indicators: A Review of Reports Currently in Use*. Conducted for The State of the USA. Wold and Associates.

TABLES B-1 AND B-2 START ON THE FOLLOWING PAGE

TABLE B-1 National Indicator Sets

	America's Health Rankings (AHR)	County Health Rankings (CHR)	Community Health Status Indicators (CHSI)
Total number of indicators	39	26	200
Purpose	The purpose of AHR is to have a comparable and comprehensive national and state measure of health and health outcomes.	The purpose of CHR is to illustrate how factors in the environment affect health outcomes, such as a person's health and longevity. CHR is a "call to action" for state and local health departments and community leaders outside the public health sector to improve community health.	The purpose of CHSI is to provide health providers and community members with local community health indicators and encourage action in improving the community's health.
Primary data sources	Public, federal sector[a]		Public, federal sector,[b] local-area data
Population-health outcome measures	**Mortality** • Premature death **Morbidity** *Quality of life* • Poor–physical-health days • Poor–mental-health days • Poor or fair health *Poor birth outcomes* • Low birth weight	**Mortality** • Premature death **Morbidity** *Health-related quality of life* • Poor or fair health • Poor–physical-health days • Poor–mental-health days *Birth outcomes* • Low birth weight	**Mortality** • All causes of death *Health-related quality of life* • Average life expectancy • Self-rated health status • Unhealthy days

Healthy People 2020 (HP2020)	State of the USA (SUSA)	Trust for America's Health (TFAH)
38 (objectives)	20	32
The purpose of HP2020 is to provide the nation with science-based, 10-year objectives for promoting health and preventing disease and in doing so to increase the population's quality of life and eliminate health disparities.	The purpose of SUSA is to assist people in tracking progress in health and health care in the United States by using high-quality statistical data and to compare the United States with other countries.	The purpose of TFAH's state data is to rank states on various public health issues and health outcomes to prevent communicable and chronic diseases and to hold officials accountable for their performance on public health issues and activities.
Public, federal sector	Public, federal sector, nonprofit sector, international[c]	Public, federal sector, nonprofit sector[d]
Morbidity • Mental health and mental disorder *Health-related quality of life* • Quality of life and well-being	**Mortality** • Infant mortality • Injury-related mortality ***Health-related quality of life*** • Life expectancy at birth • Life expectancy at 65 years old • Self-reported health status • Unhealthy days, physical and mental • Serious psychological distress	**Mortality** • Infant mortality

Continued

TABLE B-1 Continued

	America's Health Rankings (AHR)	County Health Rankings (CHR)	Community Health Status Indicators (CHSI)
Domain (or equivalent) • Community-health measures • Chronic health conditions • Social factors • Economic factors	Mortality • Infant mortality • Cardiovascular deaths • Cancer deaths • Premature deaths • Occupational fatalities Morbidity • Infectious disease Chronic disease • Stroke • High cholesterol • Hypertension • Heart attack • Coronary heart disease • Diabetes Environmental, community • Air pollution • Children in poverty • Violent crime Economic • Personal Income • Under-employment rate • Unemployment rate • Median household income	Education • *High-school graduation* • *College degrees* Employment • *Unemployment* Income • *Children in poverty* • *Income inequality* Family and social support • *Inadequate social support* • *Single-parent households* Community safety • *Violent-crime rate* Physical environment • *Air pollution: particulate-matter days* • *Air pollution: ozone days* Built Environment • *Access to health foods* • *Liquor-store density*	• Employment status • Disabled • Homicide • Motor-vehicle injury • Infant mortality[e] • Unintentional injury • Persons living below poverty[f] Chronic diseases, health problems • Diabetes • High blood pressure • Obesity • Coronary heart disease • Stroke • Cancer[g] Environmental health • Infectious diseases[h] • Toxic chemicals released annually • National air-quality standards met[i]

Healthy People 2020 (HP2020)	State of the USA (SUSA)	Trust for America's Health (TFAH)
• Maternal, infant, child health • Oral health • Social determinants of health **Chronic disease, health problems** • Arthritis, osteoporosis, chronic back pain • Blood disorders, blood safety • Cancer • Kidney disease • Diabetes • Disability, secondary conditions • Hearing, other sensory or communication disorders • Heart disease, stroke • HIV • Immunization, infectious diseases • Respiratory diseases • Sexually transmitted diseases • Vision **Environmental, community** • Educational, community-based programs • Environmental health • Family planning • Food safety • Global health • Injury, violence prevention • Occupational safety, health		Alzheimer's disease **Chronic diseases, health problems** • Cancer • Asthma: adult, percentage of high-school students • Obesity: adult, high-school students, children 10–17 years old • Hypertension • Diabetes **Communicable, infectious diseases** • West Nile virus • Tuberculosis **Sexually transmitted diseases** • AIDS: 13 years old and older, less than 13 years old • *Chlamydia* infection • Syphilis **Community** • Living in poverty • Median family Income

Continued

TABLE B-1 Continued

	America's Health Rankings (AHR)	County Health Rankings (CHR)	Community Health Status Indicators (CHSI)
Behavior domain (or equivalent)	• High-school graduation • Prevalence of smoking • Prevalence of binge drinking • Cholesterol check • Dental visit • Recent dental visit • Daily fruits and vegetables • Physical activity • Diet • Teen birth rate	**Health behavior** *Tobacco Use* • Adult smoking *Diet and exercise* • Adult obesity *Alcohol use* • Binge drinking • Motor-vehicle–crash death rate *Unsafe sex* • *Chlamydia*-infection rate • Teen birth rate	• High-school diploma • No exercise • Few fruits, vegetables • Smoking • Depression • Recent drug use
Health care domain: access, use, services, other	• Prenatal care • Preventable hospitalizations • Primary-care physicians	**Access to care** • *Uninsured adults* • *Primary-care–provider rate* **Quality care** • *Preventable hospital stays* • *Diabetic screening* • *Hospice use*	• Primary-care physicians in community • Dentists in community • Community, migrant health centers • Health-professional–shortage area **Preventive-service use** • Infectious disease[j] • Child prevention services[k] • Adult prevention services[l] • No care in first trimester

Healthy People 2020 (HP2020)	State of the USA (SUSA)	Trust for America's Health (TFAH)
• Nutrition, weight status • Physical activity, fitness • Substance abuse • Tobacco use	• Smoking • Physical activity • Excess drinking • Nutrition • Obesity • Condom use	• Tobacco smoking: adults, high-school students • Influenza vaccine rate 65 years old and older • Adult physical inactivity • Breastfeeding at 6 months • Fruit and vegetable intake
• Early, middle childhood • Genomics • Health communication, health information technology • Health care–associated infections	• Preventable hospitalizations • Childhood immunization • Health care expenditures • Insurance coverage • Unmet medical, dental, prescription-drug needs • Preventive services[m] • Chronic-disease prevalence[n]	**Access to Care** • Uninsured, total population and under age 18 years old • Immunization gap, 19–35 months old without all immunizations • Shortage of professions: primary care, mental-health care, dental care, nursing

Continued

TABLE B-1 Continued

	America's Health Rankings (AHR)	County Health Rankings (CHR)	Community Health Status Indicators (CHSI)
Other domains	Public health or other policies • Lack of health insurance • Immunization coverage • Public health funding		Birth measures • Birth weight[o] • Number of births[p] • Premature birth **Access to care** • Uninsured • Medicare • Medicaid

[a] Data sources include BRFSS; National Center for Education Statistics; Census of Fatal Occupational Injuries, Bureau of Labor Statistics; Department of Labor, Crime in the United States: 2008 Federal Bureau of Investigation; Population Survey, Mortality and Morbidity Weekly Reports, CDC; Environmental Protection Agency; Census Bureau; Trust for America's Health; National Immunization Program at CDC; American Medical Association, Physician Characteristics and Distribution in the United States; The Dartmouth Atlas of Health Care; National Heart, Lung and Blood Institute; Division for Heart Disease and Stroke Prevention, National Center for Chronic Disease Prevention and Health Promotion.

[b] Data sources include National Vital Statistics System, NCHS; BRFSS (2000–2006); Census Bureau; Healthy People 2010; Notifiable Infectious Diseases; Toxic Release Inventory Data, Environmental Protection Agency Air Quality Standards; Medicare Enrollment County Data at the Centers for Medicaid and Medicare Services; Area Resource File, Health Resources and Services Administration; American Medical Association Physician Master File; American Dental Association; State and County Demographics Report, Health Resources and Services Administration Geospatial Data Warehouse.

[c] Data sources include BRFSS; NHANES; NCHS; World Health Organization: Statistical Information System and Report on Global Tobacco Epidemic; National Survey on Drug Use and Health; Global Database on Body Mass Index; Centers for Medicaid and Medicare Services; National Health Expenditure Account, Organisation for Economic Co-operation and Development; Medical Expenditure Panel Survey; Census Bureau Current Population Survey; American Community Survey, Agency for Healthcare Research and Quality.

[d] Data sources include Census Bureau; CDC HIV/AIDS Surveillance Report; Alzheimer's Association Report; BRFSS; National Immunization Survey at CDC; American Cancer Society, HHS; CDC Division of Vector-Borne Infectious Diseases; CDC STI Disease Surveillance; NCHS; Health Resources Services Administration Geospatial Data Warehouse.

Healthy People 2020 (HP2020)	State of the USA (SUSA)	Trust for America's Health (TFAH)
• Medical-product safety • Older adults • Public health infrastructure		• Medical cost of obesity • Public health preparedness Birth Measures • Low birth weight • Premature births

e Infant-mortality indicators also broken down into white non-Hispanic, black non-Hispanic, Hispanic, neonatal, postneonatal.

f This information is broken down into age distributions (under 19 years, 19–64 years, 65–84 years, and 85+ years), race and ethnicity (white, black, American Indian, Asian/Pacific Islander, and Hispanic).

g Cancer of lung, colon, or breast.

h Cases of Escherichia coli, Salmonella, Shigella infection reported, expected per county.

i Particles of CO, NO_2, SO_2, O_3, particulate matter, lead measured.

j Cases of syphilis, congenital rubella syndrome, pertussis, measles, hepatitis A, hepatitis B, tuberculosis, influenza, AIDS reported, expected.

k Such indicators as immunizations, dental caries, prevalence of lead screening are not collected at national level and must be obtained locally.

l Percentage of population within county who had Pap smear, mammography, sigmoidoscopy, pneumonia vaccine, influenza vaccine.

m Age-appropriate services recommended by US Preventive Services Task Force and influenza vaccination.

n Diabetes, cardiovascular disease, chronic obstructive pulmonary disease, chronic bronchitis and emphysema, asthma, cancer, arthritis.

o Low birth weight, very low birth weight.

p Under 18 years old, 40–54 years old, unmarried.

SOURCES: America's Health Rankings, 2009, 2010; Community Health Status Indicators, 2009; Community Health Status Indicators Project Working Group, 2009; HHS, 2009a,b; SUSA, 2010a; Trust for America's Health, 2010.

TABLE B-2 Community Health Data Sets

	Alameda County
Total number of indicators	60
Purpose	The purpose of the Alameda County Public Health Department's report is to provide a detailed description of inequities in the economic, social, physical, and service environments affecting health and leading to death from "unnatural causes." Data and policy analysis can be used by residents to identify and advocate for policies that can reduce social and health inequalities, evaluate progress, and propose polices that affect inequities.
Primary data sources	Public sector, government[a]
Population health outcome measures	• Mortality Rate (census tract) • All causes of mortality • Self-reported health status • Life expectancy at birth

Seattle–King County	City of Saskatoon	New York City
67	31	33 (10 core)
The purpose of King County Community Indicators is to provide a broad array of comprehensive, population-based data to community-based organizations, community health centers, public agencies, policy-makers, and the general public.	The purpose of Saskatoon's community analysis is to describe the extent of health disparity, determine the causes of the health disparity, explain that most health disparity is preventable, and suggest that evidence-based policy options with sufficient public support should proceed into action.	The purpose of NYC Policy for a healthier New York is to improve the health of New Yorkers; having policy-makers, residents, communities, businesses, organizations by developing policies, laws, regulations that will improve environmental, economic, social conditions affecting health; emphasizing preventive health care, improving quality of care, expanding access to care; health promotion to inform, educate, engage residents to improve their health, health of their communities.
Public sector[b] • Life expectancy at birth • Life expectancy at age 65 years Mortality • Leading causes of death • Infant mortality Health outcomes, overall health • Fair or poor health • Years of healthy life	Public sector[c] • Infant mortality • All causes of mortality • Life expectancy at birth • Life expectancy at age 65 years • Self-rated health status[d] • Overweight or obese[e] • Physical activity[f] • Diabetes[g] • Injury hospitalization • Cardiovascular-disease death	Public sector Mortality • Deaths from smoking-related illnesses • Premature deaths from major cardiovascular disease • HIV/AIDS–related deaths • Drug overdose death (unintentional) • Colorectal-cancer death • Infant mortality[b]

Continued

TABLE B-2 Continued

	Alameda County
Domain (or equivalent) • **Community-health measures** • **Chronic health conditions** • **Community measures**	• Poverty rates • Median household income • Unemployment rates • High-school dropout rate • Neighborhood high-school graduation • Crime rate • Education level **Chronic diseases, health problems** • Asthma (children emergency-room visits) **Environmental, community** • Neighborhood poverty rate • Fast-food and convenience-store density • Density of off-sale liquor licenses • Social cohesion[i] **Transportation** • Income dedicated to transportation cost • Transit-dependent household • Public subsidies • Air quality • Annual motor-vehicle–related pedestrian injuries or deaths **Housing** • Home median sales price • Fair-market rents • Renting households under severe cost burden • Homeless service users • Homeownership rates • Housing-opportunity index • Home-loan denial • Foreclosure rate **Air quality** • Proximity to toxic-air release facilities[j]
Behavior domain	**Physical activity** • Inactivity • Place near home to walk, exercise • Safe to exercise outdoors

Seattle–King County	City of Saskatoon	New York City
• Suicide[k] • Frequent mental distress • Level of education[l] • Living in poverty **Communicable disease** • Tuberculosis incidence • Chlamydial infections • Gonorrhea • HIV/AIDS[m] **Chronic diseases** • Colorectal cancer[n] • Breast cancer[o] • Heart-disease deaths • Stroke deaths • Diabetes[p] • Asthma (adult, childhood)[q] **Physical, environmental** • Asthma (adult, childhood)[r] • Air quality · Water quality	Unemployment rate Income level Education level House price[s] Oral health **Chronic diseases, health problems** • Diabetes • Obstructive pulmonary disease • Coronary heart disease • Cerebrovascular disease • Sexually transmitted infections/HIV • Overweight or obese • Depression • Anxiety • Communicable infectious diseases[t] **Environmental, community** • Injuries, poisonings • Crime rate • Air quality • Water quality • Food access[u] • Active transportation[v]	• Preventable hospitalizations • Teen pregnancies • Education-level disparity **Chronic diseases, health problems** • Cardiovascular disease **Environmental, community** • Housing quality[w] • Neighborhood income disparity • Safety of walking, play spaces[x] • Presence of rodents[y]
• Alcohol-induced deaths • Drug-induced deaths • Smokers (adults and school age) • Overweight (adults and school age) • Obese (adults and school age) • Physical activity[z] • Drinking	• Attempted suicide • Level of physical activity[aa] • Fruit, vegetable servings • Injection-drug use • Daily smoker	• Smoking[bb] • Adult sugar consumption[cc] • Condom use in male–male sex[dd] • Alcohol hospitalizations[ee] • Fruit, vegetable servings[ff] • Obesity (adults) • Alcohol consumption (teens)[gg]

Continued

TABLE B-2 Continued

	Alameda County
Health care access, use, services, other	• Uninsured (nonelderly adult) • Uninsured person • Usual source of care • Cancer screening[hh]
Other domains	• Nativity, immigration status • Segregation[pp] • Employment health benefits • Employment by industry • Occupation • Median household income • Income level • Social support[qq] **School performance, condition** • Reading and mathematics proficiency • English level • Reading scores • School conditions • Meals[rr] • Student-reported well-being[ss] • Student-reported protective factors[tt] **Criminal justice** • Criminal rate • State-prison drug-offense admission rate • Incarceration rates under three-strikes law • County probation rate

[a] Data sources include California Health Interview Survey 2003, 2005; FBI: Uniform Crime Report; Alameda County Sheriff's Office; California Department of Finance; Alameda County Probation Department; Census Bureau 2000; California Center for Public Health Advocacy; California Department of Alcohol Beverage and Control; Environmental Protection Agency; California Department of Education; California Office of Statewide Health Planning and Development; California Highway Patrol, National Transit Database; Communities for a Better Environment; Labor Market Information System; State of cities Data System;

Seattle–King County	City of Saskatoon	New York City
• Adults with no health insurance • Children with no health insurance • Adults with unmet medical need • Childhood immunizations • Influenza vaccination (adults) • Pneumonia vaccination (adults) • Late or no prenatal care • Mammography • Dentist visit last year	• Immunizations[ii]	• Preventable hospitalizations • Medical care access[ii] • Psychological distress—no treatment[kk] • Colonoscopy[ll] • HPV vaccination[mm] Screenings • HIV-tested[nn] • Chlamydia-tested[oo]
Nativity[ww] **Overall health** • Activity limitation • Unhealthy days[xx] **Maternal, child health** • Birth weight rates[yy] • Preterm births • Maternal smoking during pregnancy **Reproductive health** • Adolescent birth rate • Adolescent pregnancy rate **Injury, violence** • Homicide • Assault • Firearms-related deaths • Motor-vehicle injuries • Motor-vehicle deaths • Suicide hospitalizations • Suicides	**Children 10–15 years old** • Self-reported health status • Depressed • Anxious • Bully comparison • Suicidal thoughts • Low self-esteem • Smoking • Alcohol use • Marijuana use	• Psychological distress—interference[zz] • Adults with hypertension needing medication and taking it • Adults with high cholesterol taking medication • Breastfeeding[aaa]

DataQuick: Foreclosures; National Association of Homebuilders, Federal Financial Institutions Examination; Department of Housing and Urban Development; American Community Survey; Department of Commerce, Bureau of Economic Analysis; Census 2000 Equal Employment Opportunity Data.

[b] Data sources include Births, deaths, abortions, hospitalizations: Washington State Department of Health, Center for Health Statistics; BRFSS, Department of Health and

Continued

TABLE B-2 Continued

Human Services, Centers for Disease Control and Prevention; Washington State Department of Health Center for Health Statistics; Seattle and King County; American Community Survey: Census Bureau; King County Community Health Survey: Public Health—Seattle and King County; State Population Survey: Washington State Office of Financial Management; Healthy Youth Survey: Washington State Department of Health; Puget Sound Clean Air Agency; Washington State Cancer Registry: Washington State Department of Health; National Immunization Survey: CDC; Population estimates: Washington State Department of Health, Vista Partnership, Krupski Consulting: Washington State Population Estimates for Public Health.

[c] Canadian Institute for Health Information (CIHI), Student health survey.

[d] Percentage of population (12+ years old) who reported their health as very good or excellent.

[e] Percentage of population (18+ years old).

[f] Percentage of population (12+ years old) who reported levels of active, moderately active, or inactive.

[g] Age-adjusted prevalence.

[h] Also have an infant-mortality disparity measure for injuries, sudden infant death syndrome.

[i] People in neighborhood can be trusted, willing to help each other, get along, share values.

[j] Broken down by demographic characteristics, population racial and ethnic composition, households living within 1 mile, public-school proximity.

[k] Hospitalizations, deaths.

[l] High-school education, bachelor's degree.

[m] Indicators for mortality, incidence, prevalence.

[n] Incidence, death.

[o] Incidence, death.

[p] Prevalence, mortality, related mortality.

[q] Prevalence, hospitalizations.

[r] Prevalence, hospitalizations.

[s] Average rental price, average vacancy rate.

[t] Norovirus, tuberculosis, pneumococcal disease, methicillin-resistant staphylococcus, West Nile virus.

[u] Food insecurity, cost of healthy eating.

[v] Walking, cycling, public transit.

[w] Poor housing quality, by neighborhood.

[x] Measured by pedestrian-injury hospitalizations of children.

[y] Measured by properties with signs of rats.

[z] CDC recommendation for adults and children, no physical activity.

[aa] Active, moderate, inactive.

[bb] Adults who currently smoke, high-school students who currently smoke.

[cc] Adults who consume an average of one or more sugar-sweetened beverages per day.

[dd] Men who have sex with men who report using a condom every time they have anal sex.

[ee] Hospitalizations for problems attributable to alcohol.

[ff] Adults eating no servings in the previous day.

[gg] High-school students who drank alcohol in preceding 30 days.

[hh] Prostatic, breast, cervical.

[ii] Preschool, school, adult, influenza, high-risk.

[jj] Adults who did not get needed medical care.

[kk] Adults with serious psychological distress who did not receive treatment.

[ll] Adults 50 years old and older who have had a colonoscopy in the last 10 years.

[mm] Girls 13–17 years old who have received vaccination.

[nn] Adults who have been tested for HIV.

[oo] Sexually active women under 26 years old.

[pp] Race or ethnicity, economic, schools.

[qq] Someone to get together with for relaxation, love and making you feel wanted, understanding problems, helping with daily chores when sick.

[rr] School free or reduced-price meal-program enrollment.

[ss] Physical fight at school, moved in last year, depression, skipped breakfast.

[tt] High expectations, caring relationship, lacks meaningful participation.

[uu] Not born in United States.

[vv] Mean number, physical and mental.

[ww] Low-birth weight singleton births, all births; very-low-birth weight singleton, all births.

[xx] Adults who have serious psychological distress that interferes with their lives or activities.

[yy] Mothers who breastfeed exclusively for at least 2 months.

[zz] Adults who have serious psychological distress that interferes with their lives or activities.

[aaa] Mothers who breastfeed exclusively for at least 2 months.

SOURCES: Alameda County Public Health Department, 2008; Saskatoon Regional Health Authority, 2007; Seattle and King County Public Health, 2010; Summers et al., 2009.

Appendix C

Meeting Agendas
Held by the Committee on Public Health
Strategies to Improve Health
(November 2009–May 2010)

Meeting One: Tuesday, November 3, 2009
National Academy of Sciences, Washington, DC

8:00 – 8:10 am   Welcome and Introductions
                   Marthe Gold
                   IOM Committee Chair

8:10 – 8:30 am   The Charge to the Committee
                   James S. Marks
                   Senior Vice President, Robert Wood Johnson
                   Foundation

8:30 – 8:45 am   Committee questions and discussion

8:45 – 9:00 am   Public Health, Prevention, and Health Care Reform
                   Georges Benjamin
                   Executive Director, American Public Health
                   Association

9:00 – 9:15 am   Committee questions and discussion

9:15 – 9:45 am   Funding for State Public Health Agencies: Status
                   and Impact
                   Paul Jarris
                   Executive Director, Association of State and
                   Territorial Health Officials

Jeffrey Engel
State Health Director, North Carolina

9:45 – 10:00 am	The Perspective of State Governments *Joyal Mulheron* *Program Director, Public Health, Health Division,* *National Governors Association*
10:00 – 10:30 am	Committee questions and discussion
10:30 – 10:40 am	Break
10:40 – 11:00 am	Public Health Perspective on Implementing Health Care Reform *Karen Hendricks* *Director of Policy Development, Trust for* *America's Health*
11:00 – 11:10 am	Committee questions and discussion
11:10 – 11:30 am	The Prevention for a Healthier America Report *Ruth Finkelstein* *Vice President for Health Policy, New York* *Academy of Medicine*
11:30 – 11:40 am	Committee questions and discussion
11:40 am – 12:10 pm	Funding for Local Public Health Agencies: Status and Impact *David Fleming* *Director and Health Officer, Seattle & King County* *Robert Pestronk* *Executive Director, National Association of County* *and City Health Officials*
12:10 – 12:30 pm	Committee questions and discussion
12:30 pm	Concluding comments and adjourn

Meeting Two: Monday, January 21, 2010
Hyatt Regency Washington, Capitol Hill, Washington, DC

8:30 – 8:40 am	Welcome and Introductions *Marthe Gold, Committee Chair, and Steven* *Teutsch, Committee Vice-Chair*
8:40 – 9:00 am	Health Indicators at the State and National Level[s]: The Wisconsin Indicators and America's Health Rankings *Patrick Remington* *Professor, Population Health Sciences* *Director, Population Health Institute, University of* *Wisconsin, Madison*
9:00 – 9:20 am	The State of the USA Indicators *George Isham (via phone)* *Member of the IOM Committee* *Medical Director and Chief Health Officer,* *HealthPartners, Inc.*
9:20 – 9:50 am	Committee questions and discussion *(Remington and Isham)*
9:50 – 10:00 am	Break
10:00 – 10:30 am	Summary Measures of Population Health: an Overview *Dennis Fryback* *Professor Emeritus, Population Health Sciences* *University of Wisconsin School of Medicine and* *Public Health*
10:30 – 11:00 am	Committee questions and discussion
11:00 – 11:30 am	A Canadian Perspective on Measuring Population Health *Michael Wolfson* *University of Ottawa* *Statistics Canada (until November 2009)*

11:30 am – 12:00 pm	National Data Sources for Measures or Indicators *Edward Sondik* *Director, National Center for Health Statistics* *Centers for Disease Control and Prevention (CDC)*
12:00 – 12:30 pm	Committee questions and discussion *(Wolfson and Sondik)*
12:30 – 1:45 pm	Lunch
1:45 – 2:15 pm	National Data Sources: BRFSS *Lina Balluz* *Chief, Surveillance Program Office, Division of* *Behavioral Surveillance, CDC*
2:15 – 2:45 pm	Committee questions and continue discussion on national data sources *(Wolfson, Sondik, Balluz)*
2:45 – 3:25 pm	Health Indicators at the State and Local Level[s] *Linda Rudolph* *Deputy Director, Center for Chronic Disease* *Prevention and Health Promotion* *California Department of Public Health* *Cory Neudorf* *Chief Medical Health Officer, Saskatoon Health* *Region, Saskatchewan, Canada*
3:25 – 4:00 pm	Committee questions and discussion *(Rudolph, Neudorf)*
4:00 – 5:00 pm	Concluding remarks and discussion
5:00 pm	Adjourn

Meeting Three: Thursday, March 4, 2010
The Beckman Center of the National Academies, Irvine, California

8:00 – 8:10 am	Welcome and Introductions *Marthe Gold, IOM Committee Chair, and Steven* *Teutsch, IOM Committee Vice-Chair*

8:10 – 8:50 am	Health Indicators *Ron Bialek* *President, Public Health Foundation*
	Committee questions and discussion
8:50 – 9:30 am	National Public Health Performance Standards *Liza Corso* *Team Leader, Office of Public Health Systems* *Performance, Office of the Chief of Public* *Health Practice, Centers for Disease Control and* *Prevention*
	Committee questions and discussion
9:30 – 10:10 am	Public Health Accreditation *Kaye Bender* *President and CEO, Public Health Accreditation* *Board*
	Committee questions and discussion
10:10 – 10:20 am	Break
10:20 – 10:40 am	Local Strategies *Jonathan Freedman* *Deputy Director, Los Angeles County Public Health*
10:40 – 11:00 am	Local Strategies *David Fleming* *Director, Seattle-King County Public Health and* *Member of IOM Committee*
11:00 – 11:30 am	Committee questions and discussion about local strategies
11:30 am – 12:30 pm	Discussion: Connecting the Dots (Performance— Accountability—Health Outcomes) *All speakers*
12:30 pm	Adjourn

Meeting Four: May 18, 2010
Keck Center of the National Academies, Washington, DC

8:00 – 8:10 am	Welcome and Introductions *Marthe Gold, IOM Committee Chair, and Steve* *Teutsch, IOM Committee Vice-Chair*
8:10 – 9:10 am	HHS Community Health Data Initiative *Todd Park, Chief Technology Officer, Department* *of Health and Human Services* *Linda Bilheimer, National Center for Health* *Statistics, Centers for Disease Control and* *Prevention (CDC)*
9:10 – 9:30 am	The Role of the Executive Branch in Public Health Law and Regulation *Mariano-Florentino (Tino) Cuéllar, Special Assistant* *to the President for Justice and Regulatory Policy,* *White House Domestic Policy Council*
9:30 – 9:50 am	Committee questions and discussion
9:50 – 10:30 am	Panel I. Authorities, Organization, and Key Issues in (and Between) Federal, State, and Local Public Health Agencies. Moderator: Lawrence Gostin, IOM Committee Member *Judith Monroe, Director, Office of State, Tribal,* *Local and Territorial Support, CDC* *Patrick Libbey, Eld Inlet Associates*
10:30 am	Break
10:40 – 11:40 am	Panel I. (Continued) *James G. Hodge, Lincoln Professor of Health* *Law and Ethics, Director, Public Health Law* *& Policy Program, University of Arizona* *Gene W. Matthews, Senior Fellow, North Carolina* *Institute for Public Health, UNC Gillings School of* *Global Public Health* *Dan Stier, Consulting Attorney, Public Health Law* *Center, William Mitchell College of Law*

11:40 am– 12:15 pm	Committee questions and discussion
12:15 pm	Lunch
1:15 – 2:15 pm	Panel II. Different Perspectives on Using the Law to Improve Population Health: Tobacco, Obesity, and Beyond. Moderator: Leslie Beitsch, IOM Committee Member. *Marice Ashe, Director, Public Health Law & Policy* *Steven D. Sugarman, Roger J. Traynor Professor of Law, University of California, Berkeley* *Scott Burris, Professor of Law, Temple School of Law*
2:15 – 2:45pm	Committee questions and discussion
2:45 pm	Break
3:00 – 4:00 pm	Panel III. Public Health Law at the Local Level. Moderator: Wilfredo Lopez, IOM Committee Member. *Wendy Perdue, Georgetown University Law Center* *Lynn Silver, Assistant Commissioner, NYC Department of Health and Mental Hygiene*
4:00 – 4:30 pm	Committee questions and discussion
4:30 – 4:45 pm	Closing comments and discussion
4:45 pm	Adjourn

Appendix D

Committee Biosketches

Marthe R. Gold MD, MPH (*Chair*), is the Logan Professor and chair of the Department of Community Health and Social Medicine of the Sophie Davis School of Biomedical Education of the City College of New York. She is a graduate of the Tufts University School of Medicine and the Columbia School of Public Health. Her clinical training is in family practice, and her clinical practice has been in urban and rural underserved settings. She served on the faculty of the University of Rochester School of Medicine from 1983 to 1990, and from 1990 to 1996 she was senior policy adviser in the Office of the Assistant Secretary for Health in the US Department of Health and Human Services (HHS). Her focus at HHS was on financing of clinical preventive services and the economics of public health programs. Dr. Gold directed the work of the Panel on Cost-Effectiveness in Health and Medicine, an expert panel whose report, issued in 1996, remains an influential guide to cost-effectiveness methods for academic and policy uses. Dr. Gold's current work is on public and decision-maker views on the use of economic analyses to inform resource-allocation decisions. She is also involved in funded initiatives that seek to increase the level of patient engagement and activation in community health-center settings. A member of the Institute of Medicine (IOM), she has contributed to a number of its reports and has served most recently on the communication collaborative of the Evidence-Based Roundtable.

Steven M. Teutsch, MD, PhD (*Vice Chair*), became the chief science officer of the Los Angeles County Department of Public Health in February 2009, where he will continue his work on evidence-based public health and policy.

He had been in the Outcomes Research and Management Program at Merck since October 1997, where he was responsible for scientific leadership in developing evidence-based clinical-management programs, conducting outcomes research studies, and improving outcomes measurement to enhance quality of care. Before joining Merck, he was director of the Division of Prevention Research and Analytic Methods (DPRAM) in the Centers for Disease Control and Prevention (CDC), where he was responsible for assessing the effectiveness, safety, and cost-effectiveness of disease and injury prevention strategies. DPRAM developed comparable methods for studies of the effectiveness and economic impact of prevention programs, provided training in the methods, developed CDC's capacity for conducting necessary studies, and provided technical assistance for conducting economic and decision analysis. The division also evaluated the effects of interventions in urban areas, developed the *Guide to Community Preventive Services*, and provided support for CDC's analytic methods. He has served as a member of the US Preventive Services Task Force, which develops the *Guide*, and on America's Health Information Community Personalized Health Care Workgroup. He currently chairs the HHS Secretary's Advisory Committee on Genetics, Health, and Society (at National Institutes of Health's [NIH's] Office of Science Policy) and serves on the Evaluation of Genomic Applications in Practice and Prevention Working Group. Dr. Teutsch received his undergraduate degree in biochemical sciences at Harvard University in 1970, an MPH in epidemiology from the University of North Carolina School of Public Health in 1973, and his MD from Duke University School of Medicine in 1974. He completed his residency training in internal medicine at Pennsylvania State University, Hershey. He was certified by the American Board of Internal Medicine in 1977 and the American Board of Preventive Medicine in 1995 and is a fellow of the American College of Physicians and the American College of Preventive Medicine. Dr. Teutsch is an adjunct professor in the Emory University School of Public Health Department of Health Policy and Management and the University of North Carolina School of Public Health. He has published over 150 articles and six books in a broad array of fields in epidemiology, including parasitic diseases, diabetes, technology assessment, health-services research, and surveillance.

Leslie Beitsch, MD, JD, is the associate dean for health affairs and directs the Center on Medicine and Public Health of Florida State University. Before joining the Florida's College of Medicine, Dr. Beitsch was Commissioner of Health for the state of Oklahoma from June 2001 to November 2003. Earlier, he had held several positions in the Florida Department of Health for 12 years, most recently as deputy secretary. He received his BA in chemistry from Emory University and his MD from Georgetown University School of Medicine and completed his internship at the Medical College of South Carolina. He received his JD from Harvard Law School.

Joyce D. K. Essien, MD, MBA, is senior advisor to the Office of the Director, Division of Partnerships and Strategic Alliances, National Center for Health Marketing, CDC; a commissioned officer with the rank of captain in the US Public Health Service at CDC; and director of the Center for Public Health Practice at the Rollins School of Public Health of Emory University. Dr. Essien leads a team in collaboration with the Sustainability Institute that is building and applying simulation and syndemic modeling applications to diabetes to inform cross-sectoral strategy, deliberation, and decision support for policy formulation and strategic interventions at the national, state, and local levels to reduce the present and future burden of diabetes. Dr. Essien was one of nine members who received the 2008 inaugural Applied Systems Thinking Award from the Applied Systems Thinking Institute for the magnitude of the problems that were being addressed (chronic-disease syndemics and health-system transformation), the interdisciplinary composition of the team, and the long track record of engagement and application in applied settings. Dr. Essien is coauthor of the *Public Health Competency Handbook—Optimizing Individual and Organizational Performance for the Public's Health* (www.populationhealthfutures.com). She serves on the Executive Committee of the Atlanta Medical Association; the boards of directors of the VHA Foundation, the Atlanta Regional Health Forum, and ZAP Asthma Consortium, Inc.; and the advisory committees for the Association for Community Health Improvement, the Association for Health Information Management Foundation, and the MPH Program at Florida A&M University, where she serves as chair. She is a member of the Bon Secours Hospital System Board Quality Committee and the Institute for Alternative Futures Biomonitoring Futures Project and Disparity Reducing Initiative. The ZAP Asthma Consortium, Inc., co-founded by Dr. Essien, is the recipient of the Rosalyn and Jimmy Carter Partnership Award (www.zapasthma.org). For her service and contributions, Dr. Essien was a recipient in 1999 of the Women in Government Award from Good Housekeeping Magazine, the Ford Foundation, and the Center for American Women and Politics at Rutgers University. She is also the recipient of the Thomas Sellars Award from the Rollins School of Public Health and the Unsung Heroine Award from Emory University. Dr. Essien is one of three recipients of the 2008 Excellence in Medicine Award from the American Medical Association Foundation.

David W. Fleming, MD, is director and health officer for Public Health in Seattle & King County, a large metropolitan health department with 2,000 employees, 39 sites, and a budget of $306 million serving a resident population of 1.9 million. Before assuming that role, Dr. Fleming directed the Bill & Melinda Gates Foundation's Global Health Strategies program, in which capacity he oversaw the foundation's portfolios in vaccine-preventable diseases, nutrition, newborn and child health, leadership, emergency relief, and cross-cutting strategies to improve access to health tools in developing countries. He is a former deputy director of CDC. Dr. Fleming has published on a wide array of public health issues and has served on multiple boards and commissions, including the board of the Global Alliance for Vaccines and Immunization. Dr. Fleming received his medical degree from the State University of New York Upstate Medical Center in Syracuse. He is board-certified in internal medicine and preventive medicine and serves on the faculty of the departments of public health at the University of Washington and Oregon Health Sciences University.

Thomas E. Getzen, PhD, is professor of risk, insurance, and health management at the Fox School of Business at Temple University and executive director of *iHEA*, the International Health Economics Association, which has 2,400 academic and professional members in 72 countries. He has also served as visiting professor at the University of Toronto, the Woodrow Wilson School of Public Policy at Princeton University, the Wharton School of the University of Pennsylvania, and the Centre for Health Economics at the University of York. His textbook *Health Economics: Fundamentals and Flow of Funds* (Wiley; 4th ed., 2010) is used in graduate and undergraduate programs throughout the world. His research focuses on the macroeconomics of health, finance, forecasting of medical expenditures and physician supply, price indexes, public health economics, and related issues. He recently completed a model of long-run medical-cost trends for use by the Society of Actuaries, building on the work of economists at the Centers for Medicare and Medicaid Services and the Congressional Budget Office.

Lawrence O. Gostin, JD, LLD (Hon.), is the Linda and Timothy O'Neill Professor of Global Health Law and the director of the O'Neill Institute for National and Global Health Law at Georgetown University. He served as the associate dean of Georgetown Law until 2008. He is also a professor at the Johns Hopkins Bloomberg School of Public Health and a visiting professor at Oxford University in the United Kingdom. He is a fellow of the Hastings Center, the Kennedy Institute of Ethics, and the Royal Society of Public Health. Professor Gostin is on the editorial boards of several journals and is law editor of the *Journal of the American Medical Association*. He directs the World Health Organization and Centers for Disease Control and Prevention Collaborating Centers on Public Health Law. Professor Gostin is a member of the IOM and has chaired four IOM committees.

Mary Mincer Hansen, RN, PhD, is director of the Masters of Public Health program and adjunct associate professor in the Department of Global Health of Des Moines University. She is the former director of the Iowa Department of Public Health in the cabinet of Governor Vilsack, where she was his designee to Governor Huckabee's National Governors Association Chair's Initiative Healthy America, which focused on addressing the obesity epidemic in America. Dr. Mincer Hansen also accompanied Governor Vilsack on his visit to China and while there met with Chinese public health leaders in Hebei Province and Beijing. In addition, she testified before the US Congress on pandemic-influenza preparedness and before the IOM's Committee on Pandemic Community Mitigation. Before being appointed as director of public health, she was an associate professor in the Drake University Department of Nursing, director of the Drake University Center for Health Issues, president of the Iowa Public Health Foundation, and a research fellow on a CDC patient-safety grant in the Iowa Department of Public Health. Dr. Mincer Hansen has served in many national positions; she has been a member of the RWJF's Advisory Committee for Partners Investing in Nursing's Future, a member of the Council of State Governments Public Health Advisory Committee, and president of the Association of State and Territorial Health Officials (ASTHO). Dr. Mincer Hansen is an appointee to the new National Health Care Workforce Commission. She also serves on the Iowa Department of Public Health Advisory Council and Senator Harkin's Nurse Advisory Committee and as president of the ASTHO Alumni Association.

George J. Isham, MD, MS, is medical director and chief health officer for HealthPartners. He is responsible for the improvement of health and quality of care and for HealthPartners research and education programs. Dr. Isham chairs the IOM Roundtable on Health Literacy. He also chaired the IOM Committee on Identifying Priority Areas for Quality Improvement and Committee on the State of the USA Health Indicators. He has served as a member of the IOM Committee on the Future of the Public's Health and on the Subcommittee on the Environment of the Committee on Quality in Health Care, which produced the reports *To Err Is Human* and *Crossing the Quality Chasm*. He has served on the Subcommittee on Performance Measures for the Committee on Redesigning Health Insurance Performance Measures, Payment and Performance Improvement Programs charged with redesigning health-insurance benefits, payment, and performance-improvement programs for Medicare. He was also a member of the IOM Board on Population Health and Public Health Practice. Dr. Isham was founding cochair of and is a member of the National Committee for Quality Assurance's Committee on Performance Measurement, which oversees the Healthcare Effectiveness Data and Information Set (HEDIS®), and he

cochairs the National Quality Forum's Advisory Committee on Prioritization of Quality Measures for Medicare. Before his current position, he was
medical director of MedCenters Health Plan in Minneapolis and in the late
1980s was executive director of University Health Care, an organization
affiliated with the University of Wisconsin–Madison.

Robert M. Kaplan, PhD, is Distinguished Professor of Health Services at
the University of California, Los Angeles (UCLA) and Distinguished Professor of Medicine at the UCLA David Geffen School of Medicine, where
he is principal investigator of the California Comparative Effectiveness
and Outcomes Improvement Center. He leads the UCLA/RAND health-
services training program and the UCLA/RAND–Centers for Disease
Control and Prevention's Prevention Research Center. He was chair of the
Department of Health Services from 2004 to 2009. From 1997 to 2004,
he was professor and chair of the Department of Family and Preventive
Medicine of the University of California, San Diego. He is a past president
of several organizations, including the American Psychological Association
Division of Health Psychology, Section J of the American Association for
the Advancement of Science (Pacific), the International Society for Quality
of Life Research, the Society for Behavioral Medicine, and the Academy of
Behavioral Medicine Research. He is a past chair of the Behavioral Science
Council of the American Thoracic Society. Dr. Kaplan is editor in chief
of *Health Psychology* and former editor in chief of *Annals of Behavioral
Medicine*. He is the author, coauthor, or editor of more than 18 books and
some 450 articles or chapters. ISI includes him in its list of the most cited
authors in the world (defined as above the 99.5th percentile). In 2005, he
was elected to the IOM.

Wilfredo Lopez, JD, graduated from the City College of New York and from
Brooklyn Law School. Mr. Lopez joined the New York City Department
of Health and Mental Hygiene as a staff attorney in 1979, became deputy
general counsel in 1980, and was appointed general counsel in 1992. In
December 2006, Mr. Lopez retired from the department and was appointed
general counsel emeritus of the department and counsel emeritus of the New
York City Board of Health. In collaboration with CDC, Mr. Lopez served
as the executive editor of "The National Action Agenda for Public Health
Legal Preparedness." He is a coeditor and coauthor of the textbook *Law in
Public Health Practice*, published by Oxford University Press. From 2007
to 2009, he spearheaded the New York City Health Code Revision Project,
the first such effort in 50 years. Since his retirement, Mr. Lopez has been a
consultant in public health and public health law.

Glen P. Mays, PhD, MPH, serves as professor and chairman of the Department of Health Policy and Management of the Fay W. Boozman College of Public Health, University of Arkansas for Medical Sciences (UAMS). He also directs the PhD program in health-systems research at UAMS. Dr. Mays's research focuses on strategies for organizing and financing public health services, preventive care, and chronic-disease management for underserved populations. He has led a series of national studies examining how public health services are organized, financed, and delivered in local communities and what factors influence the availability and quality of these services. The work has included the development of instruments and analytic techniques for measuring public health system performance and studies of the health and economic consequences of geographic variation in public health spending in the United States. He directs the Robert Wood Johnson Foundation (RWJF) Public Health Practice–Based Research Networks Program, which brings together public health agencies and researchers from around the nation to study innovations and improvements in practice. Dr. Mays's public health systems research has been funded by RWJF, CDC, the Agency for Healthcare Research and Quality, the Health Resources and Services Administration, and the National Institutes of Health and has been published in leading journals, including *Health Services Research*, *Health Affairs*, *Inquiry*, and the *American Journal of Public Health*. Dr. Mays has published more than 50 journal articles, books, and chapters on these issues. He received his PhD and MPH in health policy and administration from the University of North Carolina at Chapel Hill and completed a postdoctoral fellowship in health economics at Harvard Medical School.

Phyllis D. Meadows, PhD, MSN, RN, is associate dean for practice in the Office of Public Health Practice and clinical professor in the Department of Health Management and Policy of the University of Michigan (UM) School of Public Health, where her responsibilities include developing and teaching courses in public health administration and public health policy in the department and overseeing leadership training of public health professionals for the officee. As a senior fellow of health for the Kresge Foundation, Dr. Meadows is designing a national initiative for community health centers. Most recently, she served as director and public health officer of the City of Detroit Department of Public Health and Wellness Promotion. Before that, she spent over a decade as a program director of the W. K. Kellogg Foundation, where she worked in youth, health, health-policy, and education programming. Dr. Meadows joined the UM School of Public Health faculty in February 2009 as a clinical professor and associate director of public health practice. She holds a BS and an MS in nursing and a PhD in sociology from Wayne State University (WSU). She is the recipient of numerous honors and awards, including the WSU School of Nursing Lifetime Achievement Award, the UM Distinguished Public Health Practitioner Award, and the Michigan Department of Community Health Director's Award for Innovation in Public Health.

Poki Stewart Namkung, MD, MPH, received her AB from the University of California (UC), Berkeley; her MD from UC, Davis; and her MPH from UC, Berkeley. She is a fellow of the American College of Preventive Medicine. Dr. Namkung served as the health officer and director of public health for the city of Berkeley from 1995 to 2005 and is now the health officer and chief medical officer in the Santa Cruz County Health Services Agency. She has received many honors, including selection as a state scholar for the Public Health Leadership Institute in 1996, the California Public Health Association-North Leadership Award in 2003, and the Outstanding Berkeley Woman Award in 2005. She has served on many advisory boards and commissions and was elected president of the California Conference of Local Health Officers for 2001–2003, president of the Health Officers Association of California for 2003–2005, and president of the National Association of County and City Health Officials (NACCHO) for 2006–2007. She cochairs the Joint Public Health Informatics Taskforce, serves on NACCHO's Informatics and Immunization workgroups, and chairs the NACCHO Adolescent Health Advisory Taskforce.

Margaret E. O'Kane, MHSA, has served as president of the National Committee for Quality Assurance (NCQA), an independent nonprofit organization whose mission is to improve the quality of health care everywhere. Under Ms. O'Kane's leadership, NCQA has developed broad support among the employer and health-plan communities; today, many Fortune 100 companies will do business only with NCQA-accredited health plans. About three-fourths of the nation's largest employers use HEDIS data to evaluate the plans that serve their employees. Ms. O'Kane was named Health Person of the Year in 1996 by *Medicine & Health* magazine. She also received a 1997 Founder's Award from the American College of Medical Quality, recognizing NCQA's efforts to improve managed-care quality. In 1999, Ms. O'Kane was elected a member of the IOM. In 2000, she received CDC's Champion of Prevention award, the agency's highest honor. Ms. O'Kane began her career in health care as a respiratory therapist and went on to earn a master's degree in health administration and planning from the Johns Hopkins University.

David A. Ross, ScD, directs the Public Health Informatics Institute (PHII), a program of the Task Force for Global Health, which is affiliated with Emory University, and serves as corporate secretary of Global Health Solutions,

Inc., a nonprofit subsidiary of the Task Force. PHII supports public health practitioners in their use of information and information systems to improve community-health outcomes. He received his ScD in applied mathematics and operations research from the Johns Hopkins University. His career spans health-care research and administration, environmental-health research, and public health and medical-informatics consulting. He became the director of All Kids Count, a program of PHII supported by the RWJF, in 2000, and later began PHII, also with funding from RWJF. Dr. Ross was an executive with a private health-information systems firm, a public health service officer with CDC, and an executive of a private, nonprofit health system. In 1983, he joined CDC's National Center for Environmental Health. During his career at CDC, he worked in environmental health, CDC's executive administration, and public health practice. Dr. Ross was founding director of the Information Network for Public Health Officials, CDC's national initiative to improve the information infrastructure of public health. His research and programmatic interests reflect those of PHII: the strategic application of information technologies to improve public health practice. He served as director of the RWJF national program Common Ground and its InformationLinks national program. He served on the IOM core committee for the evaluation of the US government's global HIV/AIDS PEPFAR program and on the IOM panel recommending the research agenda for public health preparedness, is a commissioner on the Certification Commission for Health Information Technology (CCHIT), and advises the World Health Organization's Health Metrics Network Technical Working Group.

Martín José Sepúlveda, MD, FACP, is an IBM Fellow and vice president of integrated health services for the IBM Corporation. He leads a global team with responsibility for health-care policy, strategy, and design and the management system and services supporting the health and well-being of IBM's workforce and work environments. His interests and research include patient-centered primary care and medical homes, care management and coordination, total health management, workplace health promotion, risk-reduction program measurement, value-based health-care purchasing, and global occupational and health-services delivery. He is a fellow of the American College of Physicians, the American College of Occupational and Environmental Medicine, and the American College of Preventive Medicine. Dr. Sepúlveda was recently awarded honorary membership in the American Academy of Family Physicians for his work in primary-care transformation, received the 2008 John D. Thompson Distinguished Fellow Award from Yale University for Innovation in Healthcare, and received the Distinguished Alumnus Award for Professional Achievement from the University of Iowa. He serves on the IOM's Board on Population Health and Public Health Practice, the Board of Directors of the Employee Benefit Research Institute, the Board of Advisors to the School of Public Health of the University of Iowa, and the Board of the National Business Group on Health, and he chairs the Global Health Benefits Institute. He received his MD and MPH from Harvard University and completed an internal-medicine residency at the University of California, San Francisco Hospitals & Clinics, an internal-medicine fellowship at the University of Iowa Hospitals and Clinics, and an occupational-medicine residency at the National Institute for Occupational Safety and Health. He also served with the Epidemic Intelligence Service at CDC.

Steven H. Woolf, MD, MPH, is a professor in the Departments of Family Medicine, Epidemiology, and Community Health at Virginia Commonwealth University (VCU). He received his MD in 1984 from Emory University and underwent residency training in family medicine at VCU. Dr. Woolf is also a clinical epidemiologist and underwent training in preventive medicine and public health at the Johns Hopkins University, where he received his MPH in 1987. He is board-certified in family medicine and in preventive medicine and public health. Dr. Woolf has published more than 150 articles in a career that has focused on evidence-based medicine and the development of evidence-based clinical-practice guidelines, with a focus on preventive medicine, cancer screening, quality improvement, and social justice. From 1987 to 2002, he served as science adviser to and then a member of the US Preventive Services Task Force. Dr. Woolf edited the first two editions of the *Guide to Clinical Preventive Services* and is author of *Health Promotion and Disease Prevention in Clinical Practice*. He is associate editor of the *American Journal of Preventive Medicine* and served as North American editor of the *British Medical Journal*. He has consulted widely on various matters of health policy with government agencies and professional organizations in the United States and Europe and in 2001 was elected to the IOM.